Trim, athletic [...]
Dr. Steven La[...] the solution to keeping ahead in all areas of life, a medical response to the needs and concerns of Dr. Lamm's own generation. Having personally tested or followed all of the prescriptions and recommendations in this revolutionary program, Dr. Lamm makes his life-affirming practices simple to understand and manageable within the most pressured and demanding schedules. Thousands of Dr. Lamm's patients have embraced the power of Vitality Medicine, a discipline fully corroborated by the latest medical research. Now, you can discover today's secrets to success—and stay on top throughout your middle years—with

YOUNGER AT LAST

A groundbreaking program of Vitality Medicine that helps men and women maintain a competitive edge with:

- Mind-enhancing "nootropic" vitamins
- Antioxidants
- Amino acids
- Herbs
- Nonprescription supplements
- Safe, well-tested prescription medications
- Innovative strength-training techniques
- Noninvasive cosmetic treatments
- Diagnostic tests for disease prevention

L-Arginine 2g in evening (5g. hr. before)
Yohimbe 3 5.4mg. daily
Deprenyl 5 mg. 4 X per week in mornings
Trazodone 50 mg → 200 mg. daily
(desyrel) 1/2 hr. before sex or evening

**Books by Steven Lamm, M.D.
and Gerald Secor Couzens**

Thinner at Last
Younger at Last*

*Published by POCKET BOOKS

YOUNGER AT LAST

STEVEN LAMM, M.D.
AND GERALD SECOR COUZENS

POCKET BOOKS

New York   London   Toronto   Sydney   Tokyo   Singapore

No book can replace the services of a trained physician. This book is not intended to encourage treatment of illness, disease, or other medical problems by the layman. Any application of the recommendations set forth in the following pages is at the reader's discretion and sole risk. If you are under a physician's care for any condition, he or she can advise you about information described in this book.

Originally published in hardcover in 1997 by Simon & Schuster Inc.

POCKET BOOKS, a division of Simon & Schuster Inc.
1230 Avenue of the Americas, New York, NY 10020

ISBN: 0-671-02291-1

First Pocket Books printing February 1998

10 9 8 7 6 5 4 3 2 1

POCKET and colophon are registered trademarks of
Simon & Schuster Inc.

Illustrations by Timothy Jeffs
Cover design by Tai Lam Wong

Printed in the U.S.A.

To my mother, Lucy Lamm, who epitomizes Vitality Medicine. And to my wife, Kiki, who has instilled in me a sense of vitality I have never felt before. To my wonderful children, David, Suzanne, Alexandra, Morgan, and Owen: You are the reasons I need to remain younger at last.

S.L.

To Elisa, my partner in all things, and my children, Gerald, Dominic, Mary, and Rose, for their endless love and support.

G.S.C.

Contents

Preface

Two years ago, when my book *Thinner at Last* was published, it created an exciting widespread opportunity. Not only was obesity finally treated properly—with medication—as the illness it was, but it empowered patients, with their doctors' help, to correct a condition that was harming and restricting their lives.

Now, with *Younger at Last,* a brand-new age of medicine has arrived—and this time it encompasses many other facets of my patients' busy lives. Just as the *Thinner at Last* program grew out of demands to help people with weight problems, my *Younger at Last* regimen is based on requests by informed, savvy patients, solidified by medical evidence and research, to maintain their youth and vitality and to enhance it whenever possible.

My patients strive to be the best they can be, no matter what their ages. Realizing that innovations in medicine are available to them, they want to take advantage of them, right now. To them, being vital is a matter of choice.

Today, these alternatives are possible using the state-of-the-art program I have developed. I call it Vitality Medicine.

Ten years ago this book could not have been written. The science on which it is based just wasn't there; back then the concentration was on diagnosis, when a condition was already established. A decade ago, the connection between neurotransmitters and memory had not been determined; we now have prescription and nonprescription substances that will maintain and improve memory. Sexual performance was something rarely discussed between physician and patient, and physicians had little to recommend for enhancement. Today, medical science has the tools to intervene before a problem establishes itself. Or, if it shows signs of developing, we can now stop—or even reverse—it. Heart disease is less of a fear now that we finally have noninvasive tests that can alert people to early evidence of heart trouble. When it comes to skin care, revitalizing is possible with breakthrough procedures taking less than thirty minutes, and cosmeceuticals are available for maintaining and protecting skin suppleness.

We all know that aging is a part of life. But now we don't have to wait until a physical system breaks down before looking for ways to repair it. With Vitality Medicine, there are therapies available today for anyone who wants to sustain a life of good health and achievement. That means that a keen and sharp mind, a fit inner and outer body, and continued personal confidence can be yours for years longer than you thought possible.

Age is not the issue here. The issues are how we feel and how we perform. With Vitality Medicine, we can extend the gap between youth and getting older, broadening and lengthening it. With my program, you can decide how you want to give your body the boost it might need. And you can add or subtract what you want, when you require it. The potential to achieve optimal health and stamina is now in your hands. After you have read this book, I would love to hear about your experiences at my website address (http://www.youngeratlast.com) or via e-mail (YoungerAtLast @msn.com).

Welcome to the world of Vitality Medicine, where you can be *Younger at Last.*

1

Vitality Medicine:
My Prescription for Youth

Staying young is the new American dream. We live in a society that values and celebrates the attributes of youth with its energy, strength, and attractiveness. Who wouldn't want to stay that way indefinitely?

For millions of peak performers in their thirties, forties, and fifties, and even those in their sixties, this ideal presents a troubling dilemma. These men and women know that maintaining a competitive edge is key to achieving their goals, in both their private and professional lives. Experienced and savvy, tested by the rigors of jobs and families, they are used to being challenged and, despite the stress in their lives, they feel confident of themselves. Most of them take care of their bodies, exercise, and watch their diets. With several decades worth of sexual experience, they know what they like and how to attain it. Ambitious and focused, they are at the prime of their lives—and want to stay that way. Nevertheless, these men and women are keenly aware that in a world where fatigue is the enemy, faltering memory a disaster zone, and illness a pitfall to be avoided, keeping their mental and physical edges razor-sharp is the only way to sustain and live a full life.

Their dream is now a reality. Today, it's actually possible to lower age barriers, make our minds and bodies even better, and maintain that hard-won competitive edge through a combination of breakthrough medical discoveries and the aggressive use of what I call Vitality Medicine.

Vitality Medicine

Over twenty years ago, when I first began practicing medicine, my goal was simple: Make sick people well. And that's what I did, as often as possible, utilizing traditional medications and procedures. But as time went by, I began to realize that much pain and suffering could be avoided—if not eliminated—if only physicians and patients were able to head off a medical problem before it developed.

Gradually, the focus of my medical approach changed, and prevention became its key component. Soon, I began to notice a shift in my patients' attitudes. Less resigned to the inroads of disease, they began to form a combative stance against illness. The result was a partnership between us to find the most effective ways to heal. Cutting-edge diagnostics, aggressive pharmacological treatments, and the incorporation of the latest nutrition and exercise advice were our tools.

Now my patients have taken one step further. Keenly aware that they are at the peak of their lives, they want the new tools that will not only keep them mentally and physically fit—but actually better than someone twenty years younger. They want to keep what they have attained; not only do they have no intention of "going gentle into that good night"—but they have no intention of giving more of that good night to sleep than they absolutely have to!

Working with Your Doctor

As you will soon come to discover, the Vitality Medicine program is comprehensive, incorporating the best of what scientific and medical research has brought us. Vitality Medicine goes far beyond routine diet and exercise suggestions. In fact, following the suggestions outlined in the book requires not only your cooperation, but frequently the participation of your physician as well. Many aspects of this program can be fulfilled with nonprescription supplements. However, a component of Vitality Medicine involves treatment prescribed by your physician.

Ideally, you will be able to work with your current physician, since this doctor has worked with you in the past and already knows your medical history. Currently, some of you may not have a doctor or need to find a new one. In your search, you are going to come across physicians who may initially be skeptical of any medication, technique, or new technology that has not already been proven to be successful with an indisputable double-blind study. This would not be the right physician for you. The very essence of Vitality Medicine has to do with flexibility, change, and the innovative application of treatments, and a willingness to "experiment" with new drugs and techniques, knowing that they will not harm the patient, and in many cases bring about beneficial change.

What is of fundamental importance is that you find a primary-care physician who is concerned about you as an individual, who will support you in your search for answers, who will be willing to work closely with you, and even make his or her own Vitality Medicine suggestions. If possible, this should be a physician who treats the whole body, such as a family practitioner or an internist.

What the Program Can Do for You

My Vitality Medicine regimen aids men and women in their thirties through their sixties in three specific ways: It will help you:

- *feel in peak condition all of the time*
- *stay one step ahead of the competition, by maintaining mental sharpness, physical strength, and optimal performance—indefinitely*
- *look and feel ten to twenty years younger*

With Vitality Medicine, I am able to do something for my patients that was not possible before now: I can use medicine to improve vital body systems *before* they show signs of breakdown. In essence, we have the ability to:

- jump-start energy systems
- recapture and improve physical strength and endurance
- enhance memory and mental skills
- heighten sexual pleasure and enhance performance
- protect and defend the body's most vital organs, the heart and the brain
- maintain and improve the condition of the outer body and, in doing so, reflect a new inner vitality
- recontour the body, eliminating cellulite and achieving a tummy tuck—without plastic surgery

I can personally vouch for all of these exciting achievements because I have been using the program myself for the last five years. By the time I entered my forties, I noticed a very troubling phenomenon. My peers, around the same age as I was, began to exhibit very negative thoughts about aging. They looked at their parents and saw a distorted mirror image of themselves, twenty or thirty years hence. They believed that all they had worked for and achieved was about to be co-opted by someone younger. They figured that, in a very short time, their best was about to become their past.

Based heavily on a lack of medical and scientific information, and colored by cultural biases, my friends and colleagues became bogged down in the false assumption that once you get to the top of the mountain aging will inevitably pull you down. The fact is, with the right equipment, it's possible to pitch camp at that physical and mental peak indefinitely.

Peak Performance

To me, the extended period of life between thirty-five and sixty-five, even seventy, is when we ought to be at the top of our physical, mental, and creative powers. Productivity and fulfillment should be the norm; finding the next adventure or challenge should be the catalyst; awareness and action should be a constant.

Those born between 1946 and 1964, the so-called baby boomers, are now in their "peak productivity" years. Competitive and informed, they are typified by many of my patients. Consider the case of Hilary, a forty-two-year-old divorced advertising executive with a killer schedule, two teenagers, and a new serious relationship.

When Hilary's not at work she's on the cellular phone making decisions; when she's at home she has to mediate between a son and daughter who aren't, to say the least, getting along with each other. Her new beau wants time and attention, too—and his job is demanding as well. Needless to say, she wants to feel and look as good as she can, for both personal and professional reasons.

The last thing she wants is to drag herself to work after a stress-filled late night or, vice versa, to force her exhausted self to go out in the evening when she is not at her best.

When she came to see me she didn't want a quick fix. She wanted a *remedy for her life* that would ensure optimum energy, mental alertness, and as youthful and healthy an appearance as possible.

With Vitality Medicine she got just that—and continues with it to this day.

Hilary's situation is not unusual. She is one of the 76 million people born during those years whose lives are very different from past generations. They have demanding jobs that don't become easier or less time-consuming. Often it's just the opposite. Downsizing has put an enormous strain on their professional lives, where taking over more responsibilities is practically a given. Job performance is monitored daily; in today's supercompetitive world it's a constant battle to maintain a hard-won position.

Many people have two-career households where time together can be short and making the most of it is of prime importance. As caretakers, they are sandwiched between children and parents, responsible for both, as well as themselves.

Working into our seventies is no longer an option—it's a necessity for many of us today, with Social Security in possible jeopardy, traditional pensions increasingly a thing of the past, and long-term employment with a single company unlikely.

In this demanding era, the body and mind must be in optimal condition, physical strength is a requisite, and looking as terrific as you can is imperative. In today's workplace, whether it's an office, a school, a medical complex, or any of the tens of thousands of areas where we are tested daily, the person with the most stamina, energy, and vitality will win the contest.

Making the Changes

Fair or not, we all know that we are judged by how we look and act, as well as by how we perform. And, as wrong as age bias is, it exists. Therefore I find it fascinating when someone comments that utilizing the most-up-to-date medical information to provide a better life is wrong. To a number of people the idea of tinkering with nature is frightening, if not unnatural. They believe that medicine is creating a being who is less human.

Nothing could be further from the truth. How much "humanity" have we surrendered by taking vaccines that prevent horrific illnesses? Are we lessened by getting yearly checkups and monitoring our blood pressure and cholesterol levels? Are we diminished by having surgery in order to rid ourselves of a dangerous growth?

I believe we owe it to ourselves to use all that is available to allow us to be the best we can be, at every stage of our lives.

Your Second Chance at Youth

When patients ask me about how to begin, I tell all of them what I am saying in this book: Discard the tired, outdated, and inaccurate notions of how we're supposed to be at forty, fifty, or sixty. You are not your parents; you are not doomed to age the same way. We all have specific health concerns, and need to know how best they can be treated. Lifestyle, stress, and family history all play a part in the body's process of change. But we can defend ourselves against this to a remarkable degree.

One woman in her early fifties recalled a number of colds in the previous year coupled with an ever-present end-of-the-day fatigue. A man in his late thirties couldn't rid himself of the paunch he felt too young to carry around; with a family history of Type II diabetes, he was also worried that it was an early indicator of his susceptibility to the condition. Another man, in his late fifties, complained that his shoulders and knees ached. What he attributed to damp weather was actually caused by his failure to maintain his lean muscle tissue.

For all of them, less-than-perfect eating-on-the-run habits caused free-radical cell damage. Without enough fruits and vegetables, and too much fat, their bodies were more vulnerable to a host of ailments that can both speed up the aging process and threaten health.

The majority of my patients are people who want to maximize what they have achieved and keep it. While my patients' careers are greatly varied, their goal is the same: They want to take charge of their health just as they have taken charge of the other aspects of their lives. All do too much. Demanding schedules, raising (often extended) families, working on personal relationships, and high-pressure jobs mean that they do not have the time to devote to traditional, marginally effective, or untried health programs.

Instead, they seek out the wealth of new information available and act on it to keep all these aspects of themselves working perfectly.

Just as my patients are able to rid themselves of lurking

health problems while revitalizing and rejuvenating their physical and mental systems, so can you. We can literally turn back our internal clocks.

Starting the Program

My program was created to implement the principles of Vitality Medicine. Basically, there are six methods for keeping us at our most capable. The following chapters will provide in-depth information on each one.

Memory: For anyone concerned with faltering memory here are cutting-edge solutions using mind-enhancing (or nootropic) vitamins, herbs, and amino acids, as well as safe, well-tested prescription medications.

Sexual Performance: A surprise is in store for you when you read about the off-label but perfectly safe use of certain prescription medications and other potent rejuvenators. Sex is an entitlement that can be fully yours once again. And you'll be amazed to learn how exercise, an important facet of a healthy life, can, under certain conditions, actually be detrimental to sex.

Body Image: To add to my program, I have very exciting news; I will introduce you to a brand-new patented, noninvasive technique for recontouring the female and male body without surgery. A revolutionary procedure, Endermologie is for any woman wanting to rid herself of cellulite and desiring lower-body sculpting. And there are applications for men as well, such as the nonsurgical removal of "love handles." Patients are flying in from all over the world to receive this breakthrough treatment, which you'll learn about in a subsequent chapter.

Then there is aesthetic surgery, which has become so popular that it is no longer unusual—in fact, it's nearly expected. Recent technological advances can subtly eliminate visible signs of aging, making faces appear years younger while giving a psychological boost to the recipient. Recovery time, discomfort, and cost have been greatly reduced. There are innovative new treatments, such as carbon-dioxide laser surgery, a nearly bloodless procedure that can resurface the face, and vaporize wrinkles, spider veins, and age spots.

The Newest Approach to Free Radicals: Daily by-products of metabolism, oxidation, and detoxification of dangerous chemicals, these molecules, primarily derived from oxygen, are believed to contribute to human aging. Today there is a new way to fight their cell-damaging effects. Pycnogenol, an amazing new antioxidant, is an incredibly powerful natural free-radical scavenger, sixty times more efficient than Vitamin E and twenty times more potent than Vitamin C. It also offers protection against heart disease and cancer, and even blocks arthritic pain.

Running Interference with Heart Trouble: The number-one killer of American men, which is fast overtaking women as well, heart disease is a condition we all need to address. There are new twenty-first-century techniques available *now* for alerting you to the symptoms of disease years before they become apparent. While regular exercise, healthful eating, and not smoking are the most effective protections against cardiac disease, the effect of a damaging blood compound called homocysteine has emerged as a significant factor that can be made to work *for* you or *against* you. Knowing your level of this substance is even more important than keeping track of your cholesterol level. A second diagnostic test is the Ultrafast CT (computed tomography) Scan, which allows doctors to measure the amount of calcium in the coronary arteries. Researchers have found that the presence of calcium is a marker for heart disease and correlates to a high degree with the amount of atherosclerosis, or hardening of the arteries, that a person may have. A noninvasive procedure that doesn't involve inserting or injecting anything, the test shows exactly how much plaque-clogging material is in the coronary arteries. Only a few minutes long and relatively inexpensive, this test provides information that can be the single most important variable in determining how you choose to live the rest of your life.

Fighting Fatigue and Building Endurance: It's simple: If you're tired, your busy life is going to suffer. Without endurance, your longevity potential is being compromised as well. I will introduce you to an innovative strength-training program that cuts workout time by two-thirds while creating a leaner, fitter, body. And I will show how a combination of amino acids is coupled with "super proteins" to create a dynamic source of muscle-building material. The tools to combating fatigue while increasing endurance are here.

Let's Begin

Whether you are a Wall Street trader who arises before dawn each day to begin business, an attorney, sales rep, computer engineer, consultant, doctor, nurse, shopkeeper, self-employed worker, or retiree, you have a common concern: retaining your vital, competitive edge in an increasingly complex and demanding world.

In the new world of Vitality Medicine, reaching and sustaining optimal health and performance during our terrific middle years is possible.

Now, you can be younger at last.

2

Firing Up Your Memory:
Ten Medical Solutions

Today's successful men and women are unlike any others
in the past.

Not only do they handle more—they must outrun the
competition on a daily basis. Thinking at light speed, solving complex problems, leading others to the correct path
through monumental obstacles—all these are in a day's
work. Vital and healthy, they have no intention of worrying
about any potential slowing down of their mental functions.
Nor should they.

*With my Vitality Medicine program, it is possible to alter
the brain's chemistry and experience enhanced, optimal
mental function.*

Listen to Paul, a feisty forty-one-year-old who came to
see me because staying at his fiercely competitive mental
level was crucial. He arrived after he decided that hours of
studying with a memory specialist wasn't giving him the
extra edge he needed.

The head of a thriving family import-export business, it
wasn't unusual for him to juggle two international phone
calls simultaneously, sometimes in different languages.
When a new overseas competitor began putting the squeeze

on his profitability, Paul started performing double-time. Not only was he working harder and faster to keep established clients content, but he was obliged to seek out new ones to stem the ever-widening cash drain.

"Even with all the pressure I feel fine," he told me. "But I now have to write notes for myself so I don't forget anything. I need to set an alarm so I don't miss any appointments. Even so, I missed out on a big trade last week. I want something that will keep me on my toes, give me a mental leg up. My business is at stake, along with the livelihood of my employees. Not to mention my relationship with my family—it's 'our' business."

There was a simple solution to Paul's problem. I chose the prescription medication Hydergine, one that you will learn about further into this chapter and one that was able to deliver just what he needed safely and effectively.

"I've never thought so clearly," he related after taking the drug for a few weeks. "The most amazing thing is that although I'm working harder than I ever did before, I actually end up doing it in fewer hours, but with much greater results. My concentration and effectiveness—always my strong points—have increased. Best of all, I feel a lot less stressed."

Or consider Veronica's story. At forty-three and the mother of three teenagers, she worked as a supervisor of a wholesale appliance company. If that wasn't enough to fill her day, at night she took classes toward an undergraduate degree, after which she intended to start immediately an intensive three-year graduate program in speech pathology. Eventually she wanted to leave her day job to work full-time with the hearing- and speech-impaired.

"Physically, I'm terrific," she said after a checkup. "I haven't had so much as a cold in two years. But now I want to boost my brain's 'health.' Collecting and retaining information will get me where I want to go; in graduate school I'll be taking medical courses which I know will be intense. I don't want to even *think* that I won't keep up—it's just not acceptable to me. What can I do?"

Deprenyl, another prescription medication you'll learn about in this chapter, was my immediate suggestion. It was another example of a proven drug that was very widely used by physicians—but not necessarily for memory-related problems.

Receptive to the idea of a six-month trial period, she had one qualification. "I can't afford to have it slow me down at the outset, even if it picks me up later. My graduate entrance exams are coming up. I have to be at my best."

She was. Even though the test fell on the day after a weeklong sales conference, Veronica was able to pace herself so well that her study time was marked by focus, retention, and clarity. She stored an enormous reservoir of information with ease. Of the ten applicants accepted for the degree program, Veronica was at the top of the list.

Paul and Veronica are just two examples of people who are taking advantage of the choices possible in my Vitality Medicine program.

Memory Changes

Fear of future memory loss is one of the most frequent concerns voiced by my patients. Some are concerned that "they don't remember the way they used to," and "familiar faces don't trigger the corresponding names," or "important dates slip by without notice. People accuse me of not paying attention but the truth is this—I just forget."

None of these things are either unusual or indications of serious memory loss. In fact, being aware of memory lapses is a very good sign—it means that those brain systems are intact. And be reassured that they are perfectly natural, if somewhat annoying. Memory is fragile and can start to deteriorate with time. That a forty-five-year-old will need more time to process and retrieve information than a fifteen-year-old is part of being human.

Researchers believe that memory decline begins as early as age sixteen. By forty it's common to notice the first signs of memory slippage in any or all of memory's three major stages. They are:

• *Sensory memory.* This is a very brief stage in which the mind recognizes what the senses perceive. It makes the determination of just what is important and quickly transfers that data to the short-term memory.

• *Short-term memory.* Aptly named, it lasts five seconds (more or less), and can hold a maximum of seven items (a local phone number for example). Unless the details of that item are repeated continuously or written down, they will be forgotten. However, if the decision is made to remember them they will be committed to long-term memory.

• *Long-term memory.* The largest part of the memory system, this is the "bank" where meaningful information is consciously processed and recorded. Here is the storage area for thoughts, images, and experiences that go back to early childhood.

Memory occurs mainly in the hippocampus, the temporal lobes of the brain. It is here that the neurotransmitter acetylcholine is found in large quantities. As we get older, the metabolism of the brain, which burns sugar to produce energy, begins to slow down. Therefore, the power used to produce acetylcholine declines as well. Inevitably, memory problems begin to develop when the neurotransmitter supply is diminished.

Thinking Young, Today, Tomorrow, and Beyond

The key to maximizing your peak performance period—and stretching it into the years to come—is to make sure that memory, and especially retrieval capability, does not slow down. To do that, I have developed a specific program to be used right now, whether you are thirty-five, forty-five, fifty-five, or older. My plan includes the following nootropics, or brain stimulators:

• *Hydergine:* A safe and effective prescription medicine prescribed for more than two decades that may enhance the release of acetylcholine, a key neurotransmitter in the hippocampus area of the brain responsible for heightening memory. Extensively researched, Hydergine has been the subject of more than three thousand published papers, making it one of the most widely studied of all drugs. Its method of action is still unknown, but it provides an excellent response in some patients.

This is the drug that provided Paul with an extra competitive edge.

• *Deprenyl:* Another proven prescription medication introduced more than twenty years ago, this drug actively inhibits an enzyme that plays a role in brain slowdown by affecting dopamine levels in the brain.

This is the drug that helped Veronica to achieve her goals.

• *Vitamins and minerals:* Supplementation of certain substances has been shown to boost brain power. In the next few pages you will learn the dosages that work.

• *Herbal remedy:* The extract from the legendary ginkgo tree, *Ginkgo biloba* has been known to affect memory in powerful ways.

• *Amino acids:* The famous building blocks of protein play a vital role in memory by ensuring that mental acumen will not falter.

• *Site-specific nutrition:* Many foods will prompt clear mental functioning. What they are and when they should or shouldn't be eaten can make all the difference.

• *Phosphatidylserine:* Present in every cell of the body, this nutrient (also called PS) is associated with memory regulation.

• *Caffeine:* In certain quantities a morning dose of coffee or tea is a definite mental enhancer.

• *Nicotine:* Use of the transdermal patch can actually repair injured memory systems in ex-smokers. (Note: Nicotine and smoking are not the same thing.)

• *Exercise:* By stimulating the nervous system, exercise jogs memory.

Particularly appealing is the fact that my patients and I are able to tailor their programs, which are flexible and ever-changing. Based on individual responses, improvement, and special circumstances, we add and subtract components as needed. All kinds of choices are possible—and all will impart discernible benefits.

The Vitality Medicine program works for my patients, it works for me, and it will work for you, too.

The Nootropics

What exactly are nootropics? They are natural substances or chemicals that stimulate the brain. The word "nootropic" is derived from a Greek word meaning "acting on the mind." Nootropics help the brain, increasing alertness and energy as well as intensifying memory and the ability to solve problems. Influencing the ability to focus more clearly, nootropics have been found to work in two ways:

- by increasing blood flow to the brain
- by boosting the levels of one or more neurotransmitters that are believed to play a part in learning and memory

Stimulating these brain chemicals will improve brain cell metabolism and oxygen availability, giving you the means to achieve the highest level of cognition that you possibly can. (A note here: These levels differ from person to person. If you couldn't quote stock market figures after skimming the business section before taking nootropics, it's not likely you will be able to do so after taking them. What you will be able to do is strengthen the mental functions at which you already excel.)

Nootropics usually furnish results that range from subtle to startling. Overall, the uniform reactions reported to me have involved heightened focus and clarity. Reactions differ, so I'll let my patients speak for themselves:

"I was able to do a twenty-minute presentation without once referring to my notes."

"For the first time in years my wife didn't have to resort to subterfuge to remind me her birthday was around the corner."

"I love to go to the theater, but the last few years were very frustrating because I often had trouble following what was going on. Happy to say, that's now history."

"Memories I hadn't thought of in years have come back; it's like watching a home movie."

"For the first time since I was a kid everything I remember now has crystal-clear detail."

One man summed it up: "Any improvement in mental ability, big or small, gives me a leg up, and keeps me where I want—and need—to be."

The Specific Nootropics

The basic category of nootropics includes prescription medications, vitamins and minerals, amino acids, and an herbal remedy. There are two prescription medications already cited that I highly recommend: *Hydergine* and *Deprenyl*. They are the cornerstones of Vitality Medicine's memory-enhancement program.

Originally developed to treat particular medical conditions—Hydergine was used for hypertension, Deprenyl administered to sufferers of Parkinson's disease—both medications have developed an "off-label" use for memory enhancement. A very common practice, the term "off-label" means that a drug will be implemented to treat ailments other than those for which it was originally intended. In the case of Hydergine and Deprenyl, there have been off-label studies on humans to assess effects on memory, word retention, and other cognitive benefits.

Vitamins, as we know, are essential for good health, and are found in food. However, to have a therapeutic effect, supplements are necessary.

Amino acids are the "building blocks" of protein. When a food containing protein is consumed, the body first converts it to amino acids, then arranges them in thousands of different combinations that will create the specific kind of protein required to fuel almost everything we do. In the

1980s, researchers at MIT discovered what happened after protein is broken down into its component amino acids in the digestive tract. Acting on the brain, amino acids become the raw materials that ultimately affect memory, attention span, and alertness.

Ginkgo biloba is an herb that is extracted from the leaves of the similarly named tree. Employed as an herbal remedy in various cultures for more than two decades, ginkgo has been used extensively for memory enhancement.

Prescription Nootropics

Used successfully to reverse several manifestations of brain aging, some prescription medicines, particularly Hydergine and deprenyl, have demonstrated that they can improve human cognition.

As I mentioned earlier, these drugs were originally approved by the FDA for other uses. Today, however, they are often used for memory enhancement.

You should be aware, though, that each of these drugs (like all medications) has a risk/benefit profile. That is, will their potentially negative side effects bother you enough to outweigh their benefits? It's up to each individual to discuss with his or her doctor whether the merits of using the medication will counteract any of its potential risks. We'll talk about the possible side effects of each later in this chapter.

Still, if your decision is to use the drugs and find out that you tolerate them well, don't be lulled into thinking that "more is better." As with all medicines, nootropics have a bell-curve dose response. That means as you reach optimal levels you will receive the good effects; you are working your way up the curve. Take too little and, naturally, the results will be less than maximal. But take too much and the positive outcome can taper off or even lead to a worse situation—potential mental confusion or memory problems.

Determining Dosages

The recommended dosages for prescription nootropics will generally have excellent results on most people. But, since each person has a unique body chemistry, individual responses may vary. Therefore, it is in your best interest to consult with a knowledgeable physician before taking these, or any other, medications. Another good reason to talk this over with your doctor is this: The nootropic you want to take may interact badly with a medication you are already taking. Should you develop any problems after starting your nootropics, call your doctor immediately. Such interactions are common.

My patients and I find it helpful to keep a daily diary in which they can record any changes they note in memory and alertness. By alerting yourself to both positive and negative effects, you will be able to track your progress objectively.

I recommend that, whichever substance you choose, begin with the lowest recommended dosage and then slowly build up to the optimal dose. See how you feel, for a period of one to several weeks. Then consult with your doctor to determine whether it's time to increase the dosage.

The Nootropic Studies

Nootropics are all memory-enhancing agents. By increasing blood flow to the brain and the metabolism rate in mind cells, and by replacing certain brain chemicals that may have been age-depleted, nootropics can substantially improve memory. The following studies offer strong evidence:

• In Germany, in a controlled double-blind eight-week study (neither participants nor physicians knew who were given the nootropics and who took a placebo), target shooters were observed. Those who took vitamins B_1, B_6, and B_{12} performed better under competition stress than those who received the placebo.

• In Wales, a study of college students found that those given B vitamins and folate over a twelve-month period exhibited increased cognitive function.

• In Pakistan, researchers compared the difference in learning-disabled children between those taking a placebo and those taking Hydergine, the nootropic that had worked so effectively for Paul. Those taking the latter showed significant improvements in speech, comprehension, memory, and the ability to concentrate.

• Again in Germany, a double-blind clinical study revealed that large doses (600 mg) of Ginkgo biloba extract increased performance on memory tests, possibly by speeding up information retrieval from short-term memory.

• In Israel, researchers found that deprenyl, the nootropic that helped Veronica, significantly improved the memory and learning ability of elderly test animals. Canadian research in 1996 revealed similar findings in improved spatial memory tasks in older test animals.

• Research with Alzheimer's patients in Italy in 1988 found that memory was improved in all who were given phosphatidylserine (PS) for three months. This improvement was still noted for an additional three months after PS was discontinued.

• A study of eighty elderly people in France whose memory had declined proved that taking Ginkgo biloba for three months helped them perform four times better on mental aptitude tests than a control group that had been given a placebo. The most dramatic improvements were observed in short-term memory and attention span.

• Both human and animal studies have shown that a reduction in dietary boron results in a drop of alpha- and theta-brain-wave activity, a condition similar to that found in drowsy people. However, supplementation with the mineral helped increase their alertness and response time in special reaction tests.

Again and again, research has proved that nootropics will intensify the memory system. However, there used to be a time when I wasn't so sure. Like many of my colleagues, I once believed that all the nutrition we needed was accessed through the food we ate. But how many people, short on time and overburdened with responsibilities, realistically have the wherewithal to prepare and eat scientifically optimal meals that will provide even basic, much less supercharged, nutritional components?

Still, even if most people were able to feed their bodies properly from food alone (which is difficult, with so many nutrients diminished through food processing), their mental appetite would still need stoking. It's virtually impossible to ingest all the essential nutrients required in high enough quantities through your daily food intake. For one thing, many processed foods have been leeched of their natural nutrients; for another, cooking destroys valuable vitamins, even in organic produce.

I believe that the ultimate responsibility for attaining optimal nutrition rests with the individual. Whether or not the highest-quality available nutrients are ingested is a personal choice. For myself and my patients I insist on the most potent vitamin supplements.

Hydergine

Ergoloid mesylates, the drug known more commonly as Hydergine, is made from a fungus first discovered in rye fields a half century ago by Albert Hofmann (the chemist who first synthesized LSD). By affecting the dopaminergic nervous systems in the brain, Hydergine is thought to influence the production of dopamine, which controls emotions and motivation, as well as monitoring breathing, hunger, eating, sexual drive, and motor activity. In reality, however, its mechanism of action is still unknown.

Hydergine has multiple functions. By increasing protein synthesis in the brain, which is essential for memory and learning, researchers believe that it can augment cognition, perhaps by stimulating the growth of neurites, the nerve cell connections necessary to form new memories that are gradually lost during aging.

Approved by the FDA for use in treating senile dementia,

results in this area have been disappointing so far, most likely because it is often introduced too late to be of any use for patients. While of little use for the severely impaired individual, the greatest success in my practice has been with patients with mild memory complaints.

The Hydergine Effect

The reasons for Hydergine's popularity are understandable. Acting in several ways to intensify mental capabilities, it has been shown to slow down or reverse the aging process in the brain and improve memory, learning ability, and intelligence. Although its mechanism of action and overall effects are still not fully understood, researchers now believe that Hydergine acts on the brain in the following ways. It may:

- raise quantities of blood and oxygen
- increase acetylcholine levels in the hippocampus area
- increase production of the neurotransmitters dopamine and norepinephrine
- act as a powerful antioxidant that protects against free radical damage

Studies with Hydergine have noted significant improvements in a variety of cognitive functions, including alertness, memory, reaction time, abstract reasoning, and cognitive processing skill. In one study, normal volunteers who took 12 milligrams a day of Hydergine for two weeks reported improved performance in alertness as well as cognitive functions.

At forty-six, Barbara is a successful Wall Street broker who oversees multimillion-dollar deals as a way of life. When she came to see me she was already aware of the terrific effects of Hydergine—she had seen them at work in her seventy-five-year-old father.

"I can't begin to tell you the difference I see in him," she told me. "For more years than I like to admit he was losing mental ground. It was tragic to see. He had been a trial lawyer, with a reputation for incisive thinking. But then he started to deteriorate, to the point where doing a crossword puzzle was nearly impossible. Luckily, my mother took him to a new doctor, who put him on Hydergine. Now, I need to do mental gymnastics when I talk with him."

"Can a younger person use it to beef up an already strong mental state?" she asked. Absolutely, I told her. Many healthy people regularly use Hydergine to maximize mental acuity, myself included.

Barbara began a regimen and came back four months later. Ecstatic, she told me that after one month she started to notice a change. For one thing, she was no longer dependent on endless cups of coffee.

"Hydergine provides the zip coffee would give—but now it lasts all day. And that afternoon slump? It's gone. I can focus strongly throughout the day. I feel in command, and in control. And now I can keep up with my father! I feel great."

Barbara's reaction is indicative of the results I've seen with so many patients who have taken Hydergine. Confident that they will perform at peak mental efficiency, ready for any job at hand, they are sure that their mental processes will not let them down.

Since I use Hydergine to maintain peak brain function in my healthy patients, they typically build up to a maximum of 20 mg a day, taking 10 mg after breakfast and another 10 mg after lunch. Although it has no toxic side effects, Hydergine may give you a headache if you use too much too soon. Less common side effects include dizziness or light-headedness when getting up from a lying or sitting position, drowsiness, and a slow pulse. You have to find the dosage that works best for you. It is usually best to begin with a low dosage of 1 mg daily and gradually increase it. And of course you and your physician must determine the dose and timing that is right for you alone.

Deprenyl

The other prescription medication I use for memory, deprenyl, was originally developed in the 1970s by Dr. Joseph Knoll, a professor of pharmacology at the Semmelweis University of Medicine in Budapest. Also known by its generic name, selegiline, it was used to ease the symptoms of Parkinson's disease.

Deprenyl is a member of a class of drugs known as monoamine oxidase (MAO-B) inhibitors. An enzyme that plays a key role in brain deterioration, monoamine oxidase levels rise steadily as we get older, limiting neurotransmitters such as dopamine from making the crucial connections that maintain clarity and rapidity in memory and cognition. Until our late thirties, dopamine levels remain fairly stable. But by the time we reach forty-five, dopamine-containing neurons in the substantia nigra, the part of the brain that is partly responsible for the movement of our muscles, arms and legs, begin to decline. Currently, neuroscientists believe that dopamine is lost at a rate of about 13 percent per decade. However, some people exhibit a more rapid drop; if the loss approaches 30 percent of previous maximal levels Parkinson's disease results. When dopamine plummets to below 10 percent and basic functions such as respiration are lost, death is inevitable.

Deprenyl is the only medication known to selectively enhance the substantia nigra, protecting the brain's dopaminergic nervous system.

Taking deprenyl regularly after the age of forty successfully disarms monoamine oxidase, thereby slowing the age-related decrease of neurotransmitters.

Safe and Effective

It's important to differentiate between the two distinct categories of MAO inhibitors. MAO-A inhibitors, used to relieve certain types of depression, have dangerous side effects when they interact with foods containing high amounts of tyramine. Those foods include aged cheese, sausage, chicken liver, sauerkraut, and the Italian red wine Chianti. If you are taking a MAO-A inhibitor and happen to eat any of the above, you'll inevitably end up in a hospital emergency room. The combination can quickly lead to life-threatening hypertension.

Deprenyl, however, is a specific MAO-B inhibitor. Its low toxicity levels and few side effects make it an excellent choice for memory enhancement.

When Ned, an award-winning singer-songwriter in his late forties first came to see me, he complained of "brain drapes," the closing off of his creative process. Just a few years earlier, he told me, composing was a breeze.

"I'd sit down at the piano, and the notes and words would just flow from my mind to my fingers. And those songs were great; they told stories that listeners knew were the truth, for me and, I hope, for them. But now—and I can't believe I'm saying this—I feel a distinct 'block.' You know my business: you're only as popular as your last hit. I've got to get that curtain lifted—fast."

Ned began a triweekly regimen of deprenyl. Within a few months he reported dramatic changes.

"What a relief," he told me. "That medication primed my creative pump. I'm sharp, and focused on what I'm writing. The songs are coming back, day after day."

The Deprenyl Facts

An extremely safe medication, deprenyl, sold under the brand name Eldepryl, is available only by prescription in 5 mg tablets. If you have taken deprenyl in the past you must inform your physician if you experienced any unusual reactions. Also, notify your doctor if you are taking any of the following:

- the antidepressant (SSRI) medication fluoxetine (e.g., Prozac, Zoloft, Paxil)
- the weight-loss medications fenfluramine or dexfenfluramine (e.g., Pondimin, Redux)
- the narcotic pain reliever meperidine (e.g., Demerol)

I have never had any patient who has exhibited adverse reactions to deprenyl. It should be taken on an empty stomach, preferably in the morning, an hour before breakfast. To minimize any possibility of insomnia, I recommend that deprenyl not be taken any later than mid-afternoon.

Recommended Dosages and Schedules:

Age	Dose
40–50	5 mg three times a week
50–60	5 mg four times a week
60–70	5 mg every day

With the low doses recommended, side effects are extremely rare. However, you should tell your doctor immediately if you notice any adverse reactions. Possible ones include nausea, depression, insomnia, agitation, headache, migraine, constipation, or chills.

The dosage of deprenyl will, of course, differ for each patient. Your doctor will determine what that is for you. Take only as directed; do not take more of it, or for a longer period of time than has been prescribed for you.

Vitamins and Minerals That Enhance Memory

Bs for Brain Power

Take this simple test. Below is an eight-digit number. Read it once and look away, and repeat it. Then say it backwards. Here it is:

7092–3689

If either exercise is difficult you can benefit by taking more B vitamins. The body can't store them for long periods of time so Bs need to be replenished regularly. It's been known for a while that these vitamins are linked to cognitive ability, that is, memory, perception, judgment, and reasoning. They are critical for optimal brain function.

In 1995 a detailed study compared performance on memory and other mental tests with vitamin B levels in the blood. Seventy men between the ages of fifty-four and eighty-one were tested at the Jean Mayer U.S. Department of Agriculture Human Nutrition Center on Aging at Tufts

University in Boston. Researchers concluded that the men with the lowest levels of B vitamins scored much lower on cognitive tests than those with more vitamin presence.

Even more startling was the fact that men with the highest levels of homocysteine (an amino acid that erodes arteries, causing memory decline) had as poor results as people with early Alzheimer's disease. Homocysteine can accumulate in the bloodstream if there is a problem with the body's ability to convert it to cysteine, a growth-promoting amino acid, or methionine, an amino acid that aids in transporting fats to the liver. Folic acid and vitamins B_6 (pyridoxine) and B_{12} (cyanocobalamin) are critical components in this process. Inadequate intake or absorption problems can lead to elevated blood homocysteine levels.

Now it appears that homocysteine causes the same vessel damage in the brain, causing cells to self-destruct. Dr. Karen Riggs, the psychologist who directed the Tufts study, found that men with the highest homocysteine levels had poorer scores when asked to perform tests like copying a cube, a diamond, and a slanting box. While not definitive, the study strongly suggests that lack of B vitamins and folic acid will result in diminished cognitive functions.

Testing: The First Step

When a patient and I plan a nootropic program, the first step is to make sure that there are no medical problems that could be contributing to poor memory. These can include such ailments as hypothyroidism, B_{12} deficiency, (pernicious) anemia, and syphilis. I also check to see if there are any medications that may be having a negative effect (hypertensive drugs, sleep potions, and alcohol are the prime offenders). In addition to taking a routine blood test, I check thyroid function and test the patient's vitamin B_{12} levels. When the B_{12} level is low, I then try to find out if the cause is linked to diet, or else related to an abnormality in B_{12} absorption.

This was the case with Carolyn, a thirty-six-year-old interior designer. She spent a lot of time with clients, and meals with them monopolized much of her time. In order to control her calories and fat, she had adopted a strict vegan diet eschewing all meats and fish. The end result was a drain on the energy that had once sparked her to race at top speed throughout her business life.

Her tests were revealing. It turned out that her B_{12} levels were very low. The workup showed no evidence of pernicious anemia—a condition that results from the lack of *intrinsic factor,* a substance released by the lining of the stomach and needed for the absorption of vitamin B_{12}—but rather a condition entirely due to her diet. The first month I started her on 1,000 mcg of B_{12} once a week, given by injection. (A microgram [mcg] is one-thousandth of a milligram.) She also took 50 mg of B_6 three times a day. At the end of the month, her test levels showed that her B_{12} levels had risen significantly.

Carolyn and I worked together to revamp her diet and make sure that it was rich enough in nutrients to supply the energy she needed throughout her busy day. Gone were the waves of debilitating fatigue that had been slowing her down, mentally and physically.

What They Do: B_6 and B_{12}

If you are on a very strict diet without any vitamin supplementation, you may develop vitamin B deficiencies. B_6 is an extremely sensitive water-soluble vitamin which when exposed to air and heat loses its potency. As we get older, our bodies often lose their ability to use these vitamins. This means that nerve cells can't manufacture sufficient amounts of dopamine and other memory-helping chemicals.

However, this situation is easy to remedy. B_6 is found in a large selection of foods including seafood, whole grains, soybeans, wheat germ, bananas, and prunes. Include these foods in your daily diet. They will work for you, boosting your brain's long-term memory capabilities.

In addition to eating right, taking supplements can improve your memory systems. In one Dutch study, elderly men were given 20 mg doses of B_6 daily over a three-month period. They exhibited significantly improved long-term memories. *I recommend daily supplements of 20 mg—much higher than the RDA of 2 mg a day—to maintain optimal B_6 levels.*

B_{12} is another water-soluble vitamin. A crucial brain nutrient that stimulates DNA synthesis in nerve cells, B_{12} is critical for the formation of the myelin sheath that surrounds nerve cells, helping speed transmissions. Along with folic acid, its biochemical cousin, B_{12} is necessary for the manufacture of red blood cells. Any deficiency in B_{12} has unpleasant side effects: confusion, agitation, moodiness, pernicious anemia, and even diminished IQ.

However, none of these things have to happen. And if any are already present they can be reversed. Excellent sources of B_{12} are meat, fish, poultry, eggs, and milk and milk products. Note, however, that nothing that grows in the ground contains it. So, if you follow a strict vegetarian, or vegan, diet, you will likely be at risk for a B_{12} deficiency. In addition, age does play a role in B_{12}'s absorption rate and can contribute to memory loss, even if you are maintaining adequate levels of B_{12} in your diet. However, the combination of supplements with eating more B_{12}-rich foods can quickly correct these problems.

I recommend 100 mcg of B_{12} supplement a day to enhance memory and maximize cognitive abilities.

Folic Acid

Another B vitamin, folic acid (folate, folacin), both protects against heart disease and positively affects mental capacities as we grow older. Regrettably, many Americans are deficient in folic acid; it is estimated that most people take in about half the recommended 400 mcg daily.

A coenzyme that serves a vital part in the formation of DNA, the genetic material that regulates tissue processes, folic acid reduces the blood levels of homocysteine to a safe range, helping to preserve cognitive functions.

If you drink a lot of alcohol or are a woman who uses oral contraceptives, your folic acid counts may be low; both impair absorption. Low levels are linked to difficulty in concentration, depression, and several mental disorders.

Many older people with reduced presence of folic acid score lower on cognitive tests.

Folic acid is found in leafy dark-green vegetables, dried beans, whole wheat, and citrus fruits, especially orange juice. However, since not everyone will consume the quantity of foods needed daily to keep homocysteine levels in check, supplements are the solution.

I recommend a minimum of 400 mcg of folic acid supplement daily.

Vitamin E

Long heralded as the superdefender against aging, vitamin E aids in the prevention of cancer, heart disease, and artery-clogging atherosclerosis. Researchers now believe that it has remarkable memory-protection properties, too, because it guards the brain's fatty membranes against the ravages of free-radical damage. Composed of billions of highly reactive forms of oxygen made daily as a normal by-product of the body's need for energy, free radicals assault the arteries of the heart and the blood vessels of the brain. Over time this results in diminished blood flow to the brain, and can lead eventually to decreased intelligence, memory, and concentration, and even to stroke.

A recent study on the protective aspects of vitamin E was conducted at the VA Medical Center in Tucson, Arizona. It found that when mice were fed supplemental vitamin E they suffered less injury to brain-tissue proteins than did mice that didn't receive the supplementation.

A fat-soluble vitamin, E is found primarily in vegetable oils, nuts, seeds, whole grains, and wheat germ. It's also present in leafy green vegetables like kale, collards, mustard greens, and spinach. Margarine is another source; however, with recent concern over its transfatty acid content, many people are cutting back on its use. Getting enough daily vitamin E necessitates taking a supplement.

I recommend at least 400 IU (one mg equals 0.91 IU) of vitamin E supplement daily.

The Boron Boost

It has long been held that adequate levels of iodine, zinc, and iron are necessary for strong brain performance. But the relationship of other minerals, as well as their deficiency and its effect on cognition, has been poorly understood.

However, a study of the mineral boron carried out at the U.S. Department of Agriculture's Human Nutrition Research Center revealed very interesting data. It showed that people receiving 3 mg of boron daily demonstrated superior alertness, brain activity, and cognitive task performance when compared to those subjects taking only 1 mg.

When there is a deficit of boron there is a drop in alpha-wave brain activity that is associated with alertness along with an increase in theta-wave movement linked with drowsiness. Most Americans take in less than 1 mg daily, the amount contained in a medium-sized apple. According to researchers this isn't enough. This deficit can be traced to the insufficient amount of noncitrus fruits and leafy vegetables in the basic American diet. The suggested five servings of these foods every day will supply you with what you need. However, if you're not one of those people whose diets actually fulfill this daily requirement, supplementation is available. Although no Recommended Dietary Allowance has been set for boron, you should be aware that taking too much may result in kidney or reproductive system damage.

I recommend no more than 3 mg of boron supplement daily.

The Amino Acids

Tyrosine

Part of a group of neurotransmitters called catecholamines, which includes dopamine and norepinephrine, tyrosine is an amino acid with great nootropic possibilities. Whenever we are under severe mental or physical stress, excessive amounts of these neurotransmitters are released from nerve endings. If the period of siege doesn't end, the brain's communication system, vulnerable to the attack, begins to lose ground. Alertness, concentration, reaction time, and mental performance will suffer. However, extra tyrosine allows the body to rearm itself, restoring overall mental performance and mood.

Tests bear this out. Animals subjected to stress in the laboratory have been found to have reduced levels of norepinephrine. But when they were pretreated with tyrosine prior to exposure to stress, their neurotransmitter levels remained constant, and helped to build the natural store of adrenaline. Findings such as these led to human experiments. Soldiers undergoing diverse forms of stress were given tyrosine to observe its effect on their performance. In one study, soldiers, some of whom were given tyrosine and others a placebo, went into a special chamber that simulated conditions of a rapid ascent to fifteen thousand feet. Lightly clothed, the soldiers were exposed to bone-chilling cold as well as diminished oxygen supplies.

The results were impressive. The ones who took tyrosine outperformed their colleagues in a variety of mental and cognitive tests. More alert, efficient, and less anxious, they also complained less about the physical discomforts they all felt.

Tyrosine may have another beneficial effect as well. Growing clinical evidence suggests that it may be effective in treating some major forms of depression.

Readily available in food, tyrosine can be found in lean red meat, turkey, tuna, egg whites, skim milk, and legumes. Soy is a particularly good source of tyrosine (and other amino acids as well). One cup of soy milk contains four times more tyrosine than a two-ounce serving of meat or fish. Therefore, a high-protein meal will increase tyrosine levels. Nevertheless, tyrosine supplements will ensure that the correct amount is being delivered to the brain.

I recommend a supplement of 250 mg of tyrosine daily.

Choline

Related to the B vitamins, choline delivers the raw material needed for the production of acetylcholine, the neurotransmitter that plays a critical role in learning and memory. Synthesized in the body from the amino acids methionine and serine, choline is converted to acetylcholine, which enables the brain to store and retrieve facts and contributes to memory functions.

Many researchers now think that low levels of choline may actually be the cause of age-related memory loss. Research supports this view. In one study, when young, healthy subjects were given the medication scopolamine to block choline transmission in the brain, they exhibited memory problems similar to those of Alzheimer's patients. However, after they took a drug that raises choline levels their memory problems vanished.

Choline can penetrate the blood-brain barrier, which ordinarily protects the brain against daily variations in diet. Therefore, the amount of choline in a meal has a direct effect on the production of the brain's chemical signals. For instance, if you swallow a choline supplement or eat a handful of peanuts (which contain a lot of it), the choline soon passes into the blood from the digestive tract. The blood then ships it directly to the brain, where it is utilized almost immediately to make acetylcholine.

As we age, changes start to take place in the brain. Either the production of acetylcholine begins to drop or it is less efficient, which may explain forgetfulness. Adding extra choline to your diet will help to improve your memory.

Leafy green vegetables, fish, peas, beans, wheat germ, and cabbage are all good suppliers of choline, Unfortunately, its richest sources—cheese, egg yolks, and liver— are also high in cholesterol. Since many people avoid these foods for health reasons, they inadvertently set themselves up for a choline deficiency that subsequently leads to memory problems.

For it to be most effective, choline should be consumed in a pure, supplemental form. After you eat, choline and other amino acids compete with each other for access to the limited biochemical channels from blood to brain.

Therefore, it is most efficient to take choline supplements with a glass of water to keep other amino acids from contending for entry to the brain.

I recommend 350 mg of choline three times daily with meals.

Note: Before you take choline supplementation talk to your physician. Choline can produce side effects, including diarrhea. And it may aggravate manic depression in some people.

The Herbal Remedy

Ginkgo biloba

One of the most potent longevity tools, *Ginkgo biloba* is made from the pulverized leaves of the ginkgo tree. One of the world's oldest surviving organisms, ginkgos can live more than a thousand years. Its secret for incredibly long life may lie in its unfailing resistance to attacks of insects, viruses, and bacteria. In fact, the ginkgo is often planted in cities and industrial areas because of its rare ability to withstand automobile and industrial pollutants.

The healing powers of the ginkgo tree have long been known. More than five thousand years ago the Chinese used its seed and fruit to help digestion and treat various illnesses. It wasn't until the 1950s, however, that its application to memory was utilized. In Germany, after years of research on the tree's chemicals (called ginkoloids) and its distinctive double-lobed, fan-shaped leaves, scientists distilled a standardized *Ginkgo biloba* extract (GBE). Since then, millions of German prescriptions have been written for the substance, mainly to treat age-related memory problems. However, it has also been used for other conditions, including asthma, tinnitus, sexual dysfunction, and heart disorders.

How *Ginkgo biloba* Affects Memory

In the last decade, volumes of scientific papers have been published that detail animal and human experiments with *Ginkgo biloba*. All extol its ability to increase and maintain blood supply to the brain. This is a significant point: In order to function properly, the brain needs to use at least 20 percent of the total oxygen carried in the blood. With age, brain capillaries tend to stiffen and narrow, naturally limiting oxygen supply. This can lead to a number of complaints, including short-term memory problems, fatigue, headache, absentmindedness, and confusion.

Studies have shown as well that *Ginkgo biloba* aids in improving the brain's capacity to metabolize glucose (its primary fuel) into energy. In turn, this means the brain's electrical nerve cell transmissions will be fortified, leading to better memory and information processing.

Finally, research shows that *Ginkgo biloba* boosts the brain's production of ATP, the energy molecule adenosine triphosphate, as well as alpha activity, which is associated with alertness. In studies on elderly subjects, this amazing substance has been found to reinforce memory and reasoning, as well as increase the energy of the test subjects.

Nontoxic, *Ginkgo biloba* is sold in health food stores in concentrated tablet and capsule form. *I recommend one 40 mg capsule three times daily with meals.* You will likely begin to experience heightened memory within four to six weeks. To maintain those benefits continue taking the prescribed dosage.

Proper Nutrition: Feeding the Brain

As with most things, it's always helpful to get back to basics. Proper nutrition is vital to good memory function. The brain, like other organs, runs on fuel provided by what we eat. Operating on chemicals and electricity, the brain generates enough power to light a fifteen-watt bulb. As you read this page, some of the neurotransmitters, such as acetylcholine, directly affect memory and how much retention you will have. Dopamine and norepinephrine, two other neurotransmitters, influence alertness levels. The brain synthesizes these chemicals, among numerous others, from food. Therefore, what we eat plays a crucial role in maintaining mental skills. It's a simple equation: Eating right equals thinking clearly.

When a patient comes to see me, one of the first things we do is take a very close look at his or her diet. Many times, significant memory enhancement can be achieved by eliminating certain food combinations, adjusting which foods are eaten, and determining the best time of day to have them. This will ensure the release of nutrients that boost brain function when needed. I've had reports of remarkable mental changes, based on these fairly straightforward strategies.

A Warning About Fat

We know that too much fat in the diet is dangerous to physical health. Saturated fats, including all animal fats and tropical vegetable oils, can promote atherosclerosis, the progressive clogging of arteries, cancer, and other health ills. But be aware of this, too: Fatty foods slow down brain functions, impairing thinking ability, making you feel lethargic and run down. To be clearheaded and mentally sharp, you have to minimize the amount of fat you eat.

A number of studies have borne this out. In one, volunteers were injected with 360 calories of fat. Then they were instructed to concentrate on a computer screen and note whenever a zero appeared. No one was able to focus for more than three minutes. In a recent English study, high-fat and low-fat breakfasts were served to volunteers. In appearance they were identical, but the fat contents of the meals were manipulated. The high-fat meal contained 761 calories, half of them from fat. The low-fat version contained 861 calories, but only 8 percent fat. Those who ate the high-fat breakfast reported feeling sluggish, tired, and muddled for as long as three hours after eating. The low-fat eaters, on the other hand, continued to feel attentive, efficient, and energized.

Researchers now believe that the fats consumed by the body may be linked to galanin, a brain chemical produced in the hypothalamus. Activated when fats are eaten, galanin levels begin to rise, typically in the late afternoon. But the more they rise, the more fat we crave. When too much galanin is produced, you'll feel it. Common reactions are passivity, unresponsiveness, fatigue, and the inability to think clearly. Since it takes up to two or three hours for fat to be digested and get into the bloodstream, the brain doesn't receive the signal to stop eating it until it's too late, and a lot of unneeded fat has been consumed.

Therefore, the more fat you eat, the more galanin levels go up, and the more fat you crave—and store. Extra fat leads to being overweight, as well as less-than-peak performance.

Consequently, when you want your thinking to be uncluttered, limit or avoid high-fat foods, especially bacon, full-fat cheese, marbled beef, and dishes containing butter, lard, margarine, mayonnaise, and oil.

Site-Specific Nutrition

You heard it from the person who made you breakfast when you were a child, and now you're going to hear it from me, too. Eat your breakfast—it's the most important meal of the day.

It's true. In "breaking the fast" from the night before, you have the first opportunity to refuel your brain for the day, jump-starting its power. If you pass on a nutrient-rich breakfast you will also miss the chance to fill the brain with glucose. This will result in less effective concentration, coupled with that unpleasant run-down feeling that usually hits around 10:00 A.M. And a cup of coffee and a Danish will not help.

In order to achieve optimal mental levels—and positively affect your mood as well—you have to eat the right foods. Plenty of protein will deliver the biggest energy wallop. That's because protein, especially the amino acid tyrosine, makes us quick-witted and energized by helping the brain produce dopamine and norepinephrine. Once these alertness chemicals are activated, reaction time is faster and thought processes keener.

Brain boosting in the morning is easy; there is a lot of variety. Any one of these protein-rich breakfasts will give you what you need to mentally kick off the day. Some suggestions are:

- an egg-white omelet (the best protein supplier)
- a small bagel with peanut butter or tuna (hold the mayo)
- oatmeal and a cup of skim milk
- a cup of fat-free yogurt
- whole-grain high-fiber cereal and 1 cup skim milk
- 2 slices toasted whole wheat bread with 1 tablespoon of peanut butter
- protein shake (2 cups fat-free plain or vanilla yogurt blended with a banana and 3 tablespoons of wheat germ or 1 or 2 tablespoons of protein powder)

To keep your mental levels steady, lunch should also be rich in protein and low in fat. Choose meat, fish, poultry, legumes, or low-fat dairy foods, along with grains, vegetables, and fruit. Remember to have an energy-sustaining snack later in the day. Fresh fruit, peanut butter and crackers, pretzels, fig bars, and raw vegetables will do good things for your head in those hours when the "slump" starts.

Dinnertime is "down time," so plan on enjoying some carbohydrate-laden foods instead of protein, unless you must be alert at a business dinner. Pasta, rice, potatoes, and whole grains elevate serotonin levels, helping you to unwind and relax. A neurotransmitter, serotonin imparts those wonderful feelings of emotional well-being and calmness, and will help to bring you down gently after a long, hard day.

P.S.: Don't Forget Your Phosphatidylserine

Called PS, phosphatidylserine is a nutrient present in every cell of the body. It is most concentrated in brain cells and in synapses, the connections between the nerve cells. Regulating many of the proteins that have important functions in these cells, PS is especially needed for the activation of protein-kinase C, an enzyme that usually decreases with age. And PS stimulates the production of acetylcholine, the essential brain messenger involved with memory regulation.

Clinical studies have found that age-associated declines in memory, learning, and alertness seem to parallel the decline of the brain's PS levels. However, there is new evidence that PS supplementation can aid in bolstering lagging mental functions. Researchers have been conducting tests on animals with PS since the 1970s. They observed that PS increased the availability of glucose while stimulating the production of many other brain chemicals.

In 1991, a double-blind study was conducted by Dr. Thomas Crook, the former head of the National Institute of Mental Health's geriatric psychopharmacology program. PS, in 100 mg doses, was given three times a day to 140 subjects between the ages of fifty and seventy-five. All suffered from age-related memory impairment. Crook found that PS improved the cognitive age of the most impaired test subjects; their mental clocks were turned back about twelve years. Some of those participating continued to exhibit strengthened mental function for weeks after discontinuing their use of PS.

The food we eat contains insignificant amounts of PS and the body produces limited amounts. Phospholipids, a concentrated form derived from soy, are a safe and effective source. Rapidly absorbed, PS crosses the blood-brain barrier, where it appears to act exclusively in cell membranes, assisting with the generation, storage, transmission, and reception of nerve impulses.

I recommend 200 mg of PS with meals.

Caffeine

While this might surprise you, I do advocate the use of this substance in my Vitality Medicine program because caffeine does promote alertness. So go ahead and drink coffee or tea—*as long as you don't overdose on it.* Too much caffeine can sometimes raise heart rates and blood pressure excessively. Moderation is the key. (If you are one of the unusual people who doesn't need a wake-up cup in the morning, don't feel obliged to start now.)

To begin the day in top mental form, drink one or two cups of your preferred beverage—about 400 mg of caffeine—soon after awakening. A very powerful stimulant, caffeine is a naturally occurring alkaloid found in sixty-three different plant products, including coffee, cocoa beans, and tea leaves. It will perk you up, giving you a mental boost, and get you ready for the day. A mild stimulant, it starts acting on the central nervous system within a half hour of ingesting it. Caffeine inhibits certain enzymes, indirectly increasing the amount of calcium that penetrates brain cell membranes. This, in turn, increases brain activity while simultaneously decreasing the effects of any chemicals that would normally slow down brain activity.

However, more is not better, so avoid the "bottomless" cup. More than four cups of coffee or tea will have an adverse effect. Consumed in excess, caffeinated products can make a mind unfocused or foggy, and hinder performance by disrupting heart rhythm. It can also irritate the stomach lining, decrease appetite, delay sleep, cause diarrhea, and accelerate dehydration by triggering excessive excretion of urine.

Keep in mind, though, that if you decide to go without caffeine after regularly consuming high levels, withdrawal symptoms such as headache, fatigue, and drowsiness are common.

Nicotine

I am not, nor have I ever been, a proponent of smoking. As a doctor, I've seen its terrible health effects. But while I would never advocate the use of cigarettes (or cigars or pipes for that matter), new evidence about the memory-enhancing effects of nicotine impels me to add it to this chapter.

Though researchers have long known that nicotine plays an important role in improving memory, what actually happened when nicotine crossed the blood/brain barrier was a mystery. Recently, however, scientists at Columbia-Presbyterian Medical Center in New York made a discovery that may explain how nicotine heightens alertness, aiding in focus and concentration.

The results of their study show that rising nicotine levels in the brain seem to alter the signals from the central nervous system, causing nerve cells to increase their transmission of the amino acid glutamate. According to the researchers, it is this excess of glutamate that affects other cells of the nervous system, heightening awareness and helping to improve short-term memory.

This new finding apparently confirms what so many of my fellow students in medical school claimed to be a fact: Studying or taking a test was impossible without smoking. While they chalked this up to addiction, chances are that those doctors-in-training were, in fact, experiencing nicotine's glutamate effect.

I observed this in one of my patients. A two-pack-a-day smoker since he was thirteen, Henry was a partner in a law firm. Now forty-four, his perpetual hacking cough, tobacco-smelling clothes, and yellowed fingers were obvious and annoying. Additionally, his constant smoking was a concern to his new wife, who worried about his health, especially since they were contemplating starting a family.

Finally, convinced he should stop smoking, Henry started using the nicotine patch, a two-inch adhesive pad that delivers a steady dose of nicotine throughout the day. He kept using them for twelve weeks, gradually cutting back the dose over time. The patches helped him to minimize his withdrawal symptoms, namely irritability and intense cravings for cigarettes.

But while the patches, used in conjunction with behavioral therapy, helped Henry to lose his cigarette craving, he became aware of something troubling he had never before experienced. About a month after he stopped using the patches, Henry suddenly found himself struggling at work; his memory was faltering. When it was time to write legal briefs and summaries the words and ideas just weren't coming together. Were cigarettes the magic bullet that shot him full of clarity and cleverness?

Nicotine is one of the most powerful psychoactive drugs known, with addiction occurring when doses reach high levels. Smokers inhale approximately one milligram per cigarette, which quickly enters the bloodstream through the lungs, going straight to the brain. Here, it stimulates the brain, speeding up communication between cells. But by the time a cigarette is finished, the nicotine level in the blood begins to plunge, causing the body to urgently signal its need for more. Smoking a cigarette every half hour or so keeps nicotine levels elevated, but the smoker pays a devastating price.

Henry didn't want to go back to cigarettes, and in his mind he equated the patch with smoking. I explained that there was a great deal of difference between them. For one thing, the steady release of low doses of nicotine through the skin eliminates the potential for addiction. For another, the patches deliver less nicotine than cigarettes. And, most important, all the tars and poisonous gases present in smoke are eliminated. In this case, nicotine was being used as a medication to stimulate brain cells and speed up communication among them.

I pointed out that the patches delivered the nicotine his brain was used to accessing. When he discontinued the patches, he inadvertently had cut off his supply of memory booster. I once again prescribed the nicotine patch, this time at a much lower dosage. He began to take 7 mg on a Monday-to-Friday schedule, taking the patch off in the evening when he arrived home.

He reported that three hours after applying his first patch he noticed a distinct mental difference. No craving for cigarettes ever materialized. Within days he was his old self again, a fast, effective thinker.

The Best Candidates

Currently, I'm employing my nicotine treatment with patients who tried to stop smoking, but were hampered by mental disruptions, as well as ex-smokers experiencing memory problems.

Once they are smoke-free, I prescribe the 7 mg Nicotrol transdermal patch, recommending that it be used during the work week or whenever they need to perform at optimal cognition levels. Since everyone has an individualized response to nicotine, I suggest that they give the patch a test run for at least a month—put the patch on in the morning and take it off in the evening—in order to see how they respond to it. Then, based on the beneficial effects, they continue with the low-dose patch indefinitely, as needed. Research has shown that 7-mg-a-day doses are nonaddictive. None of my former smokers has either had the desire to pick up a cigarette or increase the recommended dosage. In time, many have been able to stop using the nicotine patches altogether, with some of the recommended nootropics taking their place.

Possible Side Effects

For most people there are no side effects to using the nicotine patch. But for some, discomfort is possible. In that case, it is an individual choice that is yours alone: Will the benefits outweigh the potential discomfort?

Use of the patch may affect medications you are already taking. Be sure to tell your doctor if you are taking any of the following:

- aminophylline
- insulin
- oxtriphylline
- propanolol
- propoxyphene
- theophylline

Also, if you have any illnesses, be sure to inform your physician. Tell him or her if any of the following apply to you:

- allergies to tapes or bandages
- a recent heart attack
- eczema
- high blood pressure
- insulin-dependent diabetes
- liver or kidney disease
- skipped or irregular heartbeats
- stomach ulcers
- thyroid disease

Note: The nicotine patch should not be used if you are pregnant. Human studies link miscarriages to nicotine use, while animal research has demonstrated harmful effects to the fetus.

Using the Patch

Using the patch is easy. There are five simple steps:

1. Peel the protective corner off the patch and throw the cover away.

2. Apply the patch to a dry area of skin without much oil and hair, such as the stomach, upper arm, or torso.

3. Place the silver side on the skin, pressing it firmly for ten seconds with the palm of the hand. Be sure to press around the edges of the patch.

4. Wash your hands after applying the patch.

5. Put the patch on in the morning and take it off at night. Put the next patch on in a different spot, making sure to use an alternate place each day to avoid possible skin irritation. After one week the first site may be used again.

Exercise

This last memory enhancer is just as important as the others. Like the other prescription alternatives that are based on personal choice, exercise, based on personal preference, is something that everyone needs in order to perform with superior competence.

For people who spend a lot of time sitting down, no matter how active their brains, exercise is crucial. Not only does it burn up calories, increase muscle mass (thereby providing the capacity to burn more calories), and boost metabolism, but exercise has a mental connection as well. It actually simulates the nervous system, increasing the number of electrical impulses traveling from the inner ear to the cerebellum. That means if you don't move the way you need to, cognition will be compromised. Most of my patients are aware that exercise is very important, but all complain that finding the time is a real issue.

See Chapter 7 for my innovative strength-training program that cuts traditional workout time while producing the charged, fit body that will keep you feeling and performing at your best.

New Research

We are at the dawn of a new era in brain research. Scientists around the world are working to develop new medications that will maintain and improve memory, and forestall or prevent the ravages caused by stroke and Alzheimer's disease. I'm certain that, in time, many of these new drugs, or variants of them, will eventually find their way into the Vitality Medicine program. Citicoline, a new drug developed by researchers at MIT, increases the production of acetylcholine, and has been found to have positive effects on maintaining and restoring memory. According to Paul Spiers, Ph.D., who directed much of the work on the drug, a good part of citicoline's effects are due to the fact that it helps provide cytidine, a critical substance needed to protect and keep brain neurons from deteriorating. Test results have already shown it to be very effective in helping postpone Alzheimer's disease and also in stopping and reversing brain injury caused by stroke.

"When given within forty-eight hours after suffering a stroke, citicoline dramatically limits the damage," says Spiers. "It sounds like a miracle drug, and it just may be." So impressive are the results of this drug that it is expected to receive FDA approval in 1998. While not recommended for healthy individuals, it will be interesting to see the role this drug ultimately plays in memory protection.

The hormone estrogen is another important but often overlooked memory enhancer for postmenopausal women. "Estrogen replacement is very important for maintaining short-term memory," says Dr. Frederick Naftolin, the head of Yale University's Department of Obstetrics and Gynecology and director of the Center for Research in Reproductive Biology. "Many estrogen-depleted women often complain that they're unable to remember numbers or specific tasks and need to rely on written lists."

However, these memory shortcomings often disappear when women begin estrogen replacement therapy. There is now indirect evidence that estrogen not only plays a role in maintaining memory but also in delaying Alzheimer's disease in women. "The case for estrogen replacement for women is certainly overwhelming," says Dr. Naftolin. "Not only does it offer heart and bone protection, but memory enhancement and protection as well."

There are many other factors that contribute to memory decline in addition to low estrogen levels. For both men and women, these include medication side effects (see next page), and medical or psychiatric problems such as seizure disorder, poor circulation, plaque buildup in arteries, anemia, low thyroid function, mineral deficits, Type II diabetes, and depression. Poor nutrition can also have an impact, as can long-term sleep deprivation.

Drugs That Can Hamper Memory

Many commonly prescribed and over-the-counter drugs can also affect mental sharpness and trigger short-term memory loss. They include:

- weight-loss medications (e.g., Pondimin, Redux)
- hypertension drugs (e.g., Aldomet and Inderal)
- antidepression drugs (e.g., Asendin, Elavil, Pamelor)
- antianxiety medications (e.g., Dalmane, Serax, and Valium)
- antipsychosis medications (e.g., Haldol, Mellaril, and Thorazine)
- diabetes medications (e.g., insulin)
- antacid medications (e.g., Pepcid, Tagamet, and Zantac)
- Parkinson's disease drugs (e.g., Symmetrel)

The Brain Drainers

And then there are lifestyle choices that have a negative impact on health and therefore on thinking, memory, and concentration. These brain drainers must be corrected or avoided in order for memory to function as flawlessly as possible. They are:

• *Smoking.* Although low doses of nicotine can be a potent memory enhancer, the overall effect of smoking is clearly detrimental because of its injurious effects on the lungs. Not only does smoking double your chances of suffering a heart attack, it constricts blood vessels, interfering with circulation throughout the body. When you smoke, the brain's oxygen supply is reduced, resulting in diminished mental function. Consider this, too: Once smoking destroys a brain cell it can never be regenerated.

47

• *Alcohol.* Of all the brain drainers, this is the worst. Drinking large quantities—more than two drinks a day—can inflict drastic damage to every function and organ of the body, including the brain. Additionally, alcohol burns up B vitamins, depresses brain function, can alter personality, and can upset concentration, speed of learning, and memory retrieval.

• *Obesity.* If excessive weight and body fat didn't have enough dire health effects, here is another: This condition can lead to reduced overall mental functioning. Carrying too much weight puts a great burden on the circulatory system, inhibiting the most effective employment of blood sugars, which are crucial for maximal brain functioning. Also, when obesity causes sleep apnea, a potentially life-threatening disorder that constantly disrupts sleep, cognition is adversely affected because it makes it very difficult to stay awake during the day, let alone think.

There is one more brain drainer that I list apart from the others, because, unlike its companions, it cannot be brought totally under control, and must be addressed separately:

• *Stress.* Although a part of an active, competitive life, chronic or acute stress at its worst may affect glucocorticoids, the stress hormones the body produces in times of conflict or illness. An excess of these hormones can damage brain cells and inflict attention deficit, difficulty in concentrating, and lessened short-term memory, all of which can have serious effects on your life.

Unfortunately, life can't exist without stress. Nearly all of my patients complain about stress levels, from all kinds of factors: jobs, families, relationships, financial worries, and, of course, deep concerns about changing physical attributes and mental acumen.

Working together, we have found that being aware of how pervasive stress is can be the first step to putting it in its proper place. All problems are not of equal weight, and figuring out which situation is really worth a brain drain helps to put things in perspective, often pretty quickly. It comes down to this: In order to limit the effects of stress, focus more on the various solution possibilities, rather than the problem. If it can be readily fixed or helped, it's usually not worth the negative health implications—or the mental energy.

Maintaining Memories

Even if you don't smoke, drink alcohol, or carry extra pounds, you still have a lot to juggle. Just think of all the information you have stored, in addition to the data with which you are daily bombarded. It becomes clear why recollection inevitably becomes more of a mental strain.

When John, a successful and very fit forty-seven-year-old analyst for a financial management company, sought my help he compared his mind to his computer. "It comes down to this: My competitors are younger and faster, with newer equipment. Not only do I need more RAM installed—I need an upgrade."

Good memory is one of the most significant areas of concentration for my patients and for myself. The brain is the hard drive that provides the facility to store and retrieve information, and memory is the crucial pathway to mental acuity, sharpness, and self-definition. When fully operational, it builds and maintains confidence and alertness, clearing obstacles and setting down the foundation for essential mental connections.

Summary of Nootropic Sources and Recommendations

Before starting a nootropic program, make your physician aware of your diet, and, if you are a vegan, describe several sample meals you typically prepare for yourself. Also, inform your doctor of every prescription and nonprescription item you are taking, including the daily dosages of any vitamins, minerals, and herbs you use. Make him or her aware of your daily alcohol consumption and alert them if you are taking any sleep medications.

You have many nootropic choices. I recommend that you first start with one or more of the nonprescription items. If, after a trial of several weeks, you find that these don't meet your needs, I would then switch to either Hydergine or deprenyl.

Firing Up Your Memory

Nootropic	Primary Food Source	Daily Recommendations
Hydergine	None	Begin with 1 mg and increase gradually to 20 mg; follow doctor's advice
Deprenyl	None	Age 40–50: 5 mg three times a week; 50–60: 5 mg four times a week; 60–70: 5 mg daily
Vitamin B$_6$	Seafood, whole grains, soybeans, wheat germ, bananas, prunes	20 mg daily
Vitamin B$_{12}$	Meat, fish, poultry, eggs, milk, milk products	100 mcg daily
Folic acid	Leafy green vegetables, dried beans, whole wheat, citrus fruit, orange juice	400 mcg daily
Vitamin E	Vegetable oils, nuts, seeds, whole grains, wheat germ, kale, collards, mustard greens, spinach, margarine	400 IU daily
Boron	Leafy green vegetables, noncitrus fruits	3 mg daily
Tyrosine	Lean red meat, tuna, egg whites, skim milk, legumes, soy, turkey	250 mg daily
Choline	Leafy green vegetables, fish, peas, peanuts, beans, wheat germ, cabbage, cheese, egg yolks, liver	350 mg with every meal
Ginkgo biloba	None	40 mg with every meal
Phosphatidylserine (PS)	Insignificant amounts	200 mg with every meal
Caffeine	Coffee, tea	400 mg in the morning
Nicotine	None	7 mg daily for smokers only
Estrogen	None	.625 daily for post-menopausal females only

3

Peak Sexual Performance: Today and Tomorrow

Sex. It captures our attention, sparks the imagination, and fuels our lives with satisfaction. One of life's greatest pleasures, a healthy, fulfilling sex life is an essential component of a well-rounded existence. It is a vital component of my Vitality Medicine program for this basic reason: A great sex life adds to our overall emotional, mental, and physical well-being. When sex is terrific we feel wonderful, full of vigor, and aware of ourselves in one of the best possible ways.

For today's cutting-edge man or woman an exciting sex life is not only desirable—it's essential. Having taken our right to rich, satisfying sexual experiences as a given, we understand what we like and our plan is to hold onto it. We have no intention of letting sexual desire ebb due to age, fatigue, stress, or any other factors. Nevertheless, with our lives packed so densely with the demands of work, families, and social obligations, we are now experiencing the toll that stress can take on sexual desire, frequency, pleasure, performance, and staying power.

Consistent with the goals of Vitality Medicine, the concern for my patients' well-being extends to maximizing and prolonging the sexual components of their lives. This entails addressing what is wrong, anticipating what might go amiss, enhancing what is already good, and applying new medical understanding to making it great.

Welcome to the age of scientifically investigated aphrodisiacs.

The New Aphrodisiacs: Introducing Pharmacosexology

Based on a decade of research in neuroscience, or brain chemistry, pharmacosexology deals with the effects of certain medications on sexual arousal and performance. These medications have been shown to affect brain chemistry—dopamine, noradrenergic, cholinergic, and serotonin transmitters—which, in turn, govern our sexual responses.

Neurotransmitters are chemical messengers that carry information to receptors on brain cell membranes. Some neurotransmitters can enhance sexuality; others can inhibit it. When stimulated, they therefore have the potential to increase or decrease arousal. For example, dopamine receptors typically have positive effects on sexuality. The cholinergic system also enhances sexuality, while the serotonin system, which usually inhibits, can actually, under certain chemical circumstances, stimulate sexual response. Noradrenergic neurotransmitters are normally inhibitory, reducing sexual desire.

With this understanding, scientists are targeting the sexual center of the brain in order to discover solutions for dysfunction. They are testing the actions of specific nutrients, herbs, and medications that directly influence the motivational and/or pleasure components of human sexual response. They are observing their effects on the central neurotransmitters—dopamine and serotonin—which directly impact sexuality and performance. These two brain chemicals, which transmit messages to nerve cells, are particularly affected by various sex-enhancing drugs. We are now in the age when the chemistry of sex can provide us with answers not only to what makes us tick sexually, but also to exactly which medications can make that pulse steadier and stronger.

What the Pharmacosexuals Can Do

We've all heard about the purported sexually enhancing effects of a number of various substances. For centuries, odd rituals, exotic foods, unusual herbs, and questionable potions have been employed to arouse and sustain sex.

Today the options are not only different—they work. Medications that are available now can:

- boost sex drive
- increase libido
- heighten sensory response
- enhance erections
- restore and increase vaginal secretions
- increase frequency and intensity of orgasms

Separating aphrodisiac fact from fiction became a very interesting aspect of my medical practice when many of my patients asked, with refreshing frankness, about what really worked. They expected specific answers to a lot of questions dealing with sexuality, libido, performance, and, of course, sexual pleasure and orgasm.

The truth, I told them, is that most "recognized" aphrodisiacs of the past have been minimally effective—at best.

The Vitality Medicine Aphrodisiacs

Happily, the reactions I've heard from my patients who have made use of the pharmacosexuals have run the gamut from laudatory to incredulous:

"I've always had a highly charged libido," stated Teri, a forty-two-year-old interior decorator, "but I've *never* experienced anything like this!"

"Since I've started the regimen my marriage has never been better," Edward, a forty-nine-year-old contractor told me. "My wife has become multiorgasmic, and after twenty-five years of sex we've discovered each other all over again."

"I thought extended sexual romps—the kind that went on for hours, with time-outs only for Champagne and oysters—were the stuff of romance novels. Make that fiction in general," confessed Maria, a thirty-seven-year-old costume designer. "I'm very happy to be proven wrong."

"To tell you the truth, I was getting concerned. I travel a lot, my business takes up a lot of time, and Sally is on the go, too," said Frank, a fifty-two-year-old venture capitalist. "The intimate times we have together we want to be exceptional. And now they always are."

The Pyr.5amid

The Vitality Medicine that I use includes a specific plan that rekindles, refreshes, and reenhances sexuality. Because people are unique and their wants and needs differ at various times of their lives, I've devised a kind of "sex pyramid." The most widely used substance appears first, the least utilized, last. As is always the case, you should discuss with your doctor what you want, your concerns, and what is most appropriate for your specific needs. The substances I use are:

• *L-arginine,* the mildest intervention, is an amino acid that increases libido and induces erections. It can be taken in supplement form by both men and women.

• *Yohimbe,* a prescription extract from the bark of an African tree, is an herbal remedy that increases libido and encourages erections. It is recommended for the man whose sexual performance occasionally wavers.

• *Deprenyl,* a safe and effective prescription medication, affects and protects dopamine levels, thereby increasing libido. It is an anti-aging sexual stimulant for men and women in their forties and fifties.

• *Trazodone,* a proven antidepressant prescription drug, stimulates smooth muscle relaxation, leading to erection in men but also prescribed for women who are mildly depressed and fatigued.

• *Testosterone,* a hormone that affects sex drive in both sexes, is recommended for women whose levels are low, as well as men whose blood tests reveal a deficiency.

• *Nitroglycerine,* a vasodilator ointment that enlarges smooth tissue, arteries, and veins, prompting erections, is for once-in-a-while experimentation.

Also highly recommended daily for both sexes are:

• *Sensual touch,* which raises levels of the naturally occurring neuropeptide oxytocin, thereby encouraging intimacy, bonding, and feelings of heightened emotional warmth before, during, and after sex.

• *Exercise,* which improves the cardiovascular and muscular systems, thereby positively enhancing brain-wave activity and intensified sexual response.

As is true with all the other aspects of my Vitality Medicine program, the sexual enhancement program is individualized to meet your specific needs, based on your medical history. In some cases, you will need to work with your physician to tailor your sexual enhancement plans, adding and subtracting components as needed. As you will see, I offer many options, and while everything may not be right, or even necessary, for you, each imparts discernible benefits.

It's also very important to remember that good sexual health is one aspect of a healthy life. In order for all systems to work at their optimal best, you must take care of the rest of your self. That means watching what you eat, keeping your body fat percentage low, not drinking alcohol to excess, controlling stress, and getting sufficient sleep. And, of course—not smoking.

Note: It's important to understand that the recommendations in this chapter are geared toward two groups of people: those who want to enhance their current sex lives, and those who might be experiencing some mild dysfunction due to age, overwork, or a variety of stresses.

All the suggestions are for men and women who are healthy. While there is help readily available for people with serious medical conditions, only one of those interventions is discussed in this book.

Talking About Sex with Your Physician

"Is your sex life satisfactory? Are you content with it?"

These are the questions that I routinely ask my patients. I do so because sexual health is a very accurate barometer of their overall general health. I also believe strongly that sexual satisfaction and happiness are a reasonable expectation for everyone—no matter how old.

Many of my new patients are startled when I query them. They often reply that their doctors never brought the subject up. And, unless they, the patients, had a specific or pressing sexual problem, they didn't mention it, either.

Talking about sexual matters with your doctor is an excellent example of a person taking charge of his or her health. When you see your doctor you usually aren't shy about discussing sleep patterns, any pains you might be experiencing, susceptibility to colds or flu, weight lost or gained, in fact any number of factors that affect your well-being. Holding back information about sexual concerns cheats both you and your doctor. For one, the physician won't be able to do a comprehensive checkup or offer a solution for a solvable problem. And the patient, of course, will not get the relief that might be readily available.

Keeping the lines of communication open benefits both patients and their doctors. If you're shy about discussing sex consider this: Altering sexual patterns for the better is often as simple as changing a prescription for a medication already being used. And new and better medical answers are being developed every day. Taking advantage of them means making your life better. Isn't that worth a little initial awkwardness?

This was exactly the case with Mark, a fifty-eight-year-old store owner who was happily married for fifteen years to Karen, who was forty-six. When he admitted that he and his wife hadn't had sex for over six months he figured that his inability to have an erection was a condition he just had to live with; he never considered that the cause might be a medical problem.

It's now estimated that upwards of thirty million American men suffer from impotence, with more than 80 percent of the cases caused by problems with the circulatory and neurological mechanisms that trigger erections. I told Mark that while his problem wasn't new, some solutions available to him were.

After a thorough medical evaluation, it was determined that he had a circulatory abnormality. However, there was a solution. Two weeks later his sex life was back, with the help of an injectable prescription medication called Caverject, a brand name of the blood-vessel dilator alprostadil.

Note: The first and only noninjectable medication for erectile difficulties was made available in early 1997. Called MUSE, the medication (alprostadil) is placed in the urethra (the opening at the end of the penis) with a small applicator, which causes the blood vessels to relax and an erection to begin within five minutes.

New drugs to treat impotency are currently undergoing tests on humans and the results have been extraordinary. Many will be in pill form. Preliminary studies on sildenafil, an experimental drug, has helped up to 90 percent of the impotent men who have taken it to achieve and maintain erections. Hopefully it will be available soon, under the trade name of Viagra. Another drug, phentolamine mesylate, which has been used for over forty years to treat hypertension, is currently undergoing human trials as an impotence medication. It will be submitted soon to the FDA for approval under the brand name Vasomax. It, too, will be in pill form.

The Prescription Aphrodisiacs

Human sexuality is driven by a number of factors, including complex behavior patterns and societal pressures. But interestingly enough, it is very possible that brain chemicals set sexual episodes in motion. These brain chemicals can be enhanced, maintained, and even restored with the new prescription aphrodisiacs.

The Dopamine Connection

Nestled deep in the brain stem, dopamine is the chemical messenger that makes us feel good. Recognized as a crucial element in sexual arousal, dopamine is believed to be responsible for evaluating and reacting to the innumerable sensory stimuli with which we are bombarded every day. As sensory information, via sight, smell, hearing, touch, and taste, is accessed by the brain, sensory states are produced. When you inhale the scent of flowers, savor a wonderful meal, or hear a piece of music and feel deeply satisfied, dopamine is at work.

The brain guards against dopamine's release very carefully, usually only allowing it out of the brain cell for brief moments. Moving from one brain cell to another, it plugs into keyholes called receptors, delivering its message. Once its job is finished, it backs out and is picked up by transporters, to be stored for the next time it's needed.

Normally, dopamine pulses on and off as required. In some people, though, its release is less frequent than in others. However, certain medications can help by triggering dopamine's release. The result is an elevated libido with the added bonus that the dopamine is prevented from returning to its normal "off" status for quite some time. The consequence: a mind and body ready for sex.

The Role of Serotonin

Dopamine's opposite, serotonin, is the calming neurotransmitter that has a significant effect on moods, levels of aggression, and sensitivity to pain, as well as which foods we seek and how much of them we eat. Too little serotonin can lead to imbalances affecting sleep and food consumption.

Serotonin is a complex neurotransmitter with multiple receptors, some of which may be sexually dampening while others may be sexually enhancing. Maintaining the correct balance of this brain chemical is critical for regulating both moods and sexual responsiveness.

For instance, when an antidepressant medication such as Prozac or Paxil is taken, serotonin is released by the brain and its levels, naturally, increase, producing more positive and optimistic states. But pervasive calming can have negative side effects, including dampened sexual desire or an inability to achieve orgasm.

New Uses for Known Medications

This new world of medications is actually rooted in a now-familiar term: off-label usage. As I mentioned in Chapter 2, some drugs have exhibited side effects that help patients in unexpectedly beneficial ways. So useful are they, doctors began to prescribe them for their off-label value, even though they have not received FDA approval for that particular use.

While these drugs have proven their effectiveness in intensifying libido and performance, some do cause discomfort. As is always the case, it is up to you, working with your physician, to determine whether these negative aspects outweigh the positive benefits. Each possible side effect of the drugs discussed will be covered in this chapter.

Determining Dosages

The recommended dosages in this book generally yield excellent results for most people. But because each person has a unique body chemistry, personal responses may vary. So as always, it is in your best interest to consult with a knowledgeable physician before taking these, or any other, medications. Your doctor must be supplied with the names of any medications you might be taking; there is always the chance that the new drug you want to take may not react well with them. If any problem with the new medication develops, call your doctor immediately; he or she will know best how to handle it.

As they do with all the various aspects of my program, my patients find it helpful to keep a daily diary to record changes, noting how they feel and perform. Being aware of both gratifying and unpleasant effects makes it easy to track progress objectively. I advise using this simple, personal procedure; it really helps.

I recommend that you begin with the lowest possible dosage of whichever substance you choose, and then slowly build up to the optimal dose.

For a period of one to several weeks, note how you are feeling and reacting. Then consult with your doctor to decide whether the dosage should be changed.

L-arginine

Jerry, a musician in his late thirties, was living the kind of life he had dreamed about as a teenager.

"Physically, I feel great—and my erections have been consistent," he stated to me. "But I have noticed that recently I have taken longer to get aroused. Maybe my lifestyle is taking its toll. My hours are crazy and I don't eat the way I should. I love women—and I have a revolving door of girlfriends. What can I use to maintain what I've got?"

My recommendation to him was to make sure his daily supply of L-arginine was sufficient. Because his schedule was so hectic, I prescribed a supplement.

Six months later he checked in to say that his concerns were gone. "I'm living an insane life, but everything is terrific. And if I'm satisfied with the the lift that L-arginine gives me, it pales next to the gratitude of my girlfriends."

An amino acid, L-arginine has recently been found to play a critical role in sex drive and ultimate sexual satisfaction. By making sure that you are furnishing enough L-arginine to your body, either from food or in supplement form, you will be increasing neurotransmitter production, thereby enhancing your sex life.

L-arginine is one of the essential raw materials used by the body to build protein. Like each of the other twenty-one natural amino acids, L-arginine performs specific and vital tasks in the body. It builds muscle, assists in the release of growth hormone from the pituitary gland, fights off infections, and battles cancer. A factor that helps to raise sperm count levels, it is estimated that at least half of sperm content consists of L-arginine.

In the past few years, researchers have discovered that this amino acid has a specific consequence on the production of nitric oxide (NO). Not to be confused with nitrous oxide (laughing gas), nitric oxide is turning out to be one of the most important and versatile chemical messengers responsible for normal body functioning.

The Nitric Oxide Connection

Research on nitric oxide has revealed new information on the molecule that used to be thought of as an energy source for bacteria. Within the body, nitric oxide has been found to fight infection as well as regulate blood flow. Physicians are now using it to moderate blood pressure, thereby helping to save the lives of patients with acute pulmonary hypertension. In this condition, the heart beats harder, forcing blood through narrowed blood vessels, increasing blood pressure in the process.

But the newest and most exciting research on nitric oxide has uncovered its application in male sexuality. It has been discovered recently that nitric oxide, working with L-arginine, plays the major role in the ability to have an erection. This capability is directly related to how much L-arginine, and oxygen, are available and can travel to the penis.

If you are a man who smokes (men who do are twice as likely to be impotent as nonsmokers), or suffers from hypertension, atherosclerosis, or diabetes, the likelihood of your experiencing a regular, firm erection has been greatly diminished. That's because each of these conditions either blocks or damages blood vessels, preventing L-arginine and oxygen-enriched blood from reaching the penis.

When sexual stimulation is present, the penile nerves transmit their signal, activating the enzyme nitric oxide synthase (NOS), which then converts L-arginine into NO within the penis.

The release of NO triggers the erection process. First, the corpora cavernosa, two rods of spongy tissue that run the length of the penis, are forced to relax and quickly fill with blood. Then, as the blood continues to expand the tissue, the veins that normally drain blood from the penis close off. The end result is an erection.

Experts now believe that the inability to have an erection is, in the great majority of cases, caused by poor blood flow through the penis, with an insufficient production of nitric oxide in the penis as the major culprit. By eventually discovering where nitric oxide is manufactured in the penis, and then developing an effective method to stimulate its release on demand, researchers hope to finally solve this problem.

The L-arginine Facts

In order to maximize daily stores of L-arginine, thereby ensuring optimal sexual responsiveness, you must be sure to take in sufficient sources of this amino acid every day. Excellent high-quality protein sources include soy, brown rice, raisins, chicken, turkey, dairy products, sesame seeds, and nuts. L-arginine supplements are also a solid investment toward maintaining and augmenting healthy sexual function.

I recommend that you take 2 g in the evening. Some of my patients have reported good results by upping their supplementation to 5 grams taken forty-five minutes to an hour before a sexual encounter.

L-arginine is a very safe substance with few side effects. However, if you have had a herpes infection and are planning on taking supplements, speak with your doctor before doing so. I recommend that all of my patients with this history also take 1 gram of lysine. The reason is this: The herpes virus in your body will utilize the extra L-arginine, providing material for replication, and hence an outbreak. The lysine will prevent this from happening.

Yohimbe

Arthur, a very successful computer software salesman was, at forty-three, someone who knew what he wanted, when he wanted it.

"I want to be very clear about this," he told me directly. "I just got married for the first time last year. My wife and I had a great sex life before we got married but in the last few months my performance just hasn't been consistent. Is there something 'natural' that I can do about it?"

One of the first questions I always ask my male patients who inquire about improving their sexual response is "Do you wake up with an erection?" The presence of a firm morning erection almost always rules out any severe physiologic problems involving decreased blood flow to the penis or hormonal problems.

Arthur was healthy and still had morning erections. Since he was taking L-arginine already, we discussed a substance that particularly intrigued him: yohimbe. An herb obtained from the inner bark of the yohimbeh, an evergreen tree that grows in Africa, it is found in Cameroon, Congo, and Gabon. Long considered an aphrodisiac by Africans, yohimbe has been used by many urologists for treating impotence. Yohimbe has been found to block the brain's noradrenergic neurotransmitters that decrease sexual impulse.

While it can take up to three weeks before there are noticeable results, yohimbe can make good sex even better for men with no sexual problems. It has the ability to heighten libido, strengthen erections, and trigger more powerful orgasms.

Arthur decided to try it. Four weeks later he told me, "I felt some mild queasiness the first few days, but that passed quickly. By week three I had the proof I needed. I felt a tingling in my lower back that was like a rocket being fueled. That was the beginning of an experience that shows no sign of ending. All our systems are go."

The Yohimbe Effect

The active ingredient of yohimbe bark is yohimbine, an alkaloid that causes an increase in small-blood-vessel dilation. This enlargement of blood vessels increases blood flow to the penis, leading to an erection. The unusual effect of yohimbe on duration of erections is due to its blocking the release of neurotransmitters that prevent penile arteries from enlarging.

Animal studies have confirmed yohimbe's sexual effects, both in sexually active and (previously) inactive animals. Widely used throughout the world, yohimbe is very popular. Men who have been given yohimbe intravenously have developed erections almost immediately. Interestingly enough, when yohimbe is injected directly into the penis erections don't occur. This apparent contradiction has led some researchers to speculate that yohimbe is possibly affecting the pleasure centers in the brain, and dopamine in particular. It may also be influencing blood levels of norepinephrine, a neurotransmitter that stimulates the sex center located in the hypothalamus. To date, however, no studies have been done on yohimbe's effect on women.

The Yohimbe Facts

I recommend three 5.4 mg tablets daily, taken morning, noon, and night. Generally well-tolerated, yohimbe can, in some instances, cause one or more of the following side effects: dizziness, nervousness, anxiety, headaches, and muscle cramps. Varying from mild to unpleasant, these symptoms often fade over time. However, should you experience any side effects, immediately contact your physician.

Although Yohimbe is available by prescription, it is also widely available in health food stores. Since there is little regulation within the health food industry, the quality of some products may be suspect. Stick with well-established companies.

Deprenyl

When Nancy, a forty-eight-year-old college professor, came for a checkup, the vibrant redhead was clearly thrilled.

"Phil and I are reveling in a very good relationship—you know he's ten years younger than I am," she confided. "I love Phil; we share the same interests and he's wonderfully attentive to me. For the first time since my divorce five years ago I feel energized and ready for anything. My kids are away at college, I'm working, and I'm taking the best care of myself that is possible. I feel sexy—and I want to stay that way.

"I love sex with Phil, just as he does with me. My only concern is that I won't be able to keep up with him. Is there a sex 'booster' I can take that will keep my sex drive in high gear?" she asked.

I told her there was a possible solution. By taking the prescription medication deprenyl she could boost her libido. I explained that although its primary use was in the treatment of Parkinson's disease, it had a stirring sexual effect for which I recommended it to my healthy patients. Taken in low dosages several times a week it is a significant sex enhancer.

Nancy was willing to give it a try. Two months later she reported that she felt an awakening of sexual feelings that were completely new to her. "I can tell you that I have a sexual energy that I never thought existed. Frankly, I always thought my libido was pretty adequate. Now I surprise myself. Phil and I are ecstatic; sex has become something to be enjoyed and anticipated. We're always looking forward to our next time."

The Deprenyl Effect

As I related in Chapter 2, my initial interest in deprenyl arose from the question of whether it could aid memory.

According to studies done at the University of Toronto, deprenyl protects against the loss of dopamine, the key neurotransmitter responsible for cognition. Most of the dopamine we have is located in a tiny area of the brain called the substantia nigra. Of all the brain cells, neurons found there age more quickly and die sooner than cells in other locations. Deprenyl goes directly to this area, helping to prevent the death of dopamine-producing neurons.

Research done in 1980, which focused on deprenyl's effect on depression, revealed another effect of the drug. In an American study in which twelve men and women found relief from depression, an unexpected side effect was observed: All the test subjects reported a heightened libido. This could be explained in two ways. First, deprenyl affects the brain's dopaminergic system, which is critical to sexual function. And second, the lifting of these patients' depression by itself permitted them to think actively about sex.

Similar prosexual effects have been noted in octogenarian patients who are given levodopa (L-dopa), another medicine used to treat Parkinson's disease. L-dopa also protects dopamine.

Dr. Joseph Knoll, the Hungarian physician and pharmacologist who is responsible for much of the developmental work on deprenyl, believes that the dopaminergic system is heavily linked to sexual functioning. In extensive research on animals, Knoll found that animals given deprenyl, even much older specimens whose sex lives were just about nonexistent, responded to the medication. Once their dormant sexual urges were reawakened, Knoll noted that they were ready to "surmount every obstacle, even if life were in the balance, to reach a sexual partner."

The research convinced me that deprenyl could have a superlative impact on the lives of my patients. When I prescribe it to those who request a "sex boost," I hear reactions that are nothing short of astounding. deprenyl has been able to:

- enliven the sex life of a forty-five-year-old woman who had recently married a man a dozen years her junior

- turn on the sexual night-light of a forty-four-year-old man who worked sixty hours a week
- awaken the sexual longing in a fifty-one-year-old man who hadn't touched his partner intimately in more than a year
- intensify the orgasms of a fifty-two-year-old woman who remarried after ten years of being divorced
- increase the number of weekly orgasms of a fifty-four-year-old man who worried that his prowess was on the decline
- jump-start the sex life of a long-married couple who worried that sex was becoming less of a pleasure and more of a chore

The Deprenyl Facts

Safe and effective, deprenyl is available by prescription only. Sold under the trade name Eldepryl, it comes in 5 mg tablets. Your physician must be informed if you ever took deprenyl and experienced any unpleasant reactions. Make sure you tell your doctor if you are currently using any of the following :

- the antidepressant fluoxetine (e.g., Paxil, Prozac, Zoloft)
- the weight-loss medications fenfluramine or dexfenfluramine (e.g., Pondimin, Redux)
- the narcotic pain reliever meperidine (e.g., Demerol)

Deprenyl should be taken an hour before breakfast, insuring an empty stomach. I advise not taking it any later than midafternoon to avoid any possibility of insomnia.

Here are my recommended dosages and schedules:

Age	Dose
40–50	5 mg three times a week
50–60	5 mg four times a week
60–70	5 mg every day

Side effects are rare because the dosages are so low. Still, your doctor should be notified as soon as any unusual reactions are experienced. Nausea, depression, insomnia, agitation, headache, migraine, constipation, or chills might occur.

Because every person is different, dosages will vary. Your physician is the best judge for deciding what will work for you. Use only as prescribed and do not take more, or for a longer period than has been recommended.

Trazodone

When Benjamin, at forty-nine a contentedly married bank executive caught up in a takeover bid, came to see me, he was troubled.

"The long hours at work are wiping me out," he related. "My grown kids are having financial problems, and I'm bailing them out. By the time I get home and have a quick dinner all I want to do is to fall into bed—to sleep. The long days and constant pressure are bringing me down and I'm always dragging. But my sleep is disrupted; I toss and turn a lot and I'm often awake at four o'clock in the morning. When I get up I feel more tired than I did the night before.

"You know that Carol works, too. We're like those two ships passing in the night; so much fog seems to be separating us. I love Carol, and I'm pleased when she initiates sex. The problem is, my brain says yes, but the rest of me is saying no. Of course this concerns me. A lot. But now Carol thinks I'm not interested in her anymore, which certainly isn't true. Is there some medical problem? I don't want to live the rest of my life this way."

Benjamin's situation wasn't unusual, and I told him so. Rewarding sex lives don't just happen, even if the two people involved care for each other deeply. Good sex, like good relationships, requires work. Because his intense work atmosphere and long hours weren't likely to change, at least in the near future, he had to take charge of the rest of his life.

I had one immediate suggestion: putting aside time for the two of them to spend together each week. Whether it was an evening out or a weekend in the country (without calls from the children), the two of them needed to devote time to their relationship. I told him that these interludes would help to clear that fog, and remind both of them of the very things they found so attractive in each other.

I suspected, too, that he may have a mild case of depression, which was something he had not verbalized. I asked him if he wanted to try a trial period with trazodone, a prescription medication whose common brand name is Desyrel. While it is used primarily as an antidepressant, I explained that I often used it in cases like Benjamin's. Trazodone reduces stress and anxiety levels and heightens sex drive. I further explained that although trazodone affects the brain's serotonin levels, it is unlike any other selective serotonin re-uptake inhibitor (SSRI) because it promotes profound sexual effects. Most antidepressant drugs in this class inhibit sexual response.

Benjamin decided to take trazodone on a trial basis.

A month later he reported back to me. "You were right; making time for just the two of us has been great. We both needed it more than we knew. But the trazodone has been terrific. I take it in the evening, about 45 minutes before a sexual encounter. I'm sleeping better and feel much less tired. And that mild depression has lifted. But the best thing is that not only has my desire increased—so has the duration of my erections. I can't begin to describe our sex life now. We thought we were hot at thirty—little did we know."

The Trazodone Effect

Benjamin is just one of many of my patients whose sex lives have been helped through trazodone. For people with histories of sexual dissatisfaction, the changes can be spectacular: It has meant the beginning of a truly satisfying sex life. For others, whose relations are compatible and exciting, there is a lift to an unbelievable level. I've been told that trazodone:

- created a whole new sex life for a subdued couple in their forties who had a less than stimulating existence together

- provided a solution for a thirty-eight-year-old man who was less interested in sex than he wanted to be due to problems on the job
- elevated the confidence and spirits of a forty-three-year-old woman whose sex life had been merely adequate before and was now sensational

The Trazodone Facts

When I prescribe trazodone tablets to my healthy patients to enhance their sexual function, I typically have them start out at 50 mg daily. This is a much lower dose than the 150 to 200 mg usually prescribed to treat depression. Of course, this dosage may be increased or decreased by your doctor, as needed.

As is the case with all medications, common side effects and precautions associated with trazodone will vary greatly from one person to the next. Since trazodone affects the serotonin neurotransmitters, it will add to the effects of excessive alcohol and other central nervous system depressants such as allergy or hay fever medications, sedatives, and sleeping aids. Check with your doctor before taking any of these drugs once you begin using trazodone.

Trazodone may lead to increased sleepiness. I recommend that it be taken a half hour before your sexual encounter, in the evening, thereby enhancing both your sex drive and improving your sleep. Like many other medications, trazodone may cause mild mouth dryness. If you experience this, chew sugarless gum and drink plenty of water throughout the day.

Note: A rare side effect is priapism, a persistent erection. If you sustain a prolonged and painful erection stop using the drug and contact your physician immediately.

Testosterone

When Richard, a fifty-four-year-old engineer, first noticed the progressive decline of his sex life, he quickly brought it to my attention.

"I'm losing my urge to have sex," he told me, not a little

incredulously. "But I guess it's inevitable," he continued, "although I have to say that I'm not happy about it. At all."

I told him that while it is true that testosterone production declines slowly with age, the process takes a while. But it's also determined by nature that quantities will drop: By age sixty-five, more than 60 percent of men have low testosterone levels.

Richard's blood test results supported what I expected. His level measured a low 310, out of a typically normal range of between 300 and 1,000 nanograms per deciliter (ng/dl) of blood. After checking for evidence of abnormalities that could be contributing to his low levels—testicular or prostate cancer, pituitary disease, or cirrhosis of the liver are known culprits—and finding none, I recommended that he have a testosterone injection.

Research at the St. Louis University Medical School has found that giving men an injectable form of this hormone for three months increases their sex drive as well as boosting muscle strength. And a study conducted in 1995 at the Chicago Medical School found that a low dose of testosterone taken for two years seemed to cause no side effects at all. According to a researcher involved with the study, the men receiving the injections felt better and had denser bones, lower cholesterol, and a greater sexual appetite than men who weren't getting the extra hormone.

With this information in hand, Richard agreed to be given an injection of 200 mg of testosterone. A few days later he called to report that his libido had been stirred. After two more weeks, he received a second shot, and soon afterwards I switched him to prescription transdermal patches. Now he could easily self-medicate without the necessity of office visits. Each night he placed two testosterone patches on his body; the thigh, upper arm, back, and abdomen are suitable sites. Each 2.5 mg patch gradually releases the hormone through the skin and into the bloodstream. In doing so, the daily rhythm of testosterone present in younger men is duplicated. After a month of using the patch, Richard called me again.

"I feel like my best sexual self. It's like I'm thirty-five again, with all systems intact."

The Role of Testosterone

Technically, testosterone is an androgen, a masculinizing hormone that directs development of muscle tissue, lowering of the voice, and overall growth. It has other applications as well, as it affects libido, memory, and lean body mass. Interestingly, at birth, boys have the same testosterone levels as young adult males. The levels do drop quickly, however, and remain low until puberty, when they rise, setting in motion masculine characteristics. Hormone production continues to climb as boys get older, tapering off at around the age of forty.

But insufficient blood levels of the hormone, a condition described as testosterone deficiency, can be caused by a number of problems and is not unusual. It is estimated to affect as many of 20 percent of men over the age of fifty. Major causes are :

- decreased activity in the pituitary gland, hypothalamus, or testes
- chronic disease, such as AIDS, diabetes, or kidney failure
- diminished testosterone production due to aging

These conditions can lead to symptoms that include diminished libido, loss of energy, decrease in bone and muscle mass, increased body fat, dry skin, and depression.

Over the past few years I have been able to address these problems by *recommending regular injections of 200 mg of testosterone followed up with the daily use of 2.5 mg transdermal patches*. The effects have been uniformly remarkable, with all the men involved reporting that their dormant sex lives have been reawakened.

Note: The long-term effects of testosterone supplementation on healthy males are still not known, and may not be for years to come. Currently, there are some medical concerns. For instance, extra testosterone may cause prostate growth, a risk for men with an already enlarged prostate, or undetected cancer in that organ. I monitor all my patients closely, and, to date, none of them has experienced these serious side effects.

Testosterone and Women

When Margaret came to see me she was, at forty-eight, already exhibiting signs of menopause. But that wasn't what brought her to my office.

"A change of life doesn't really bother me that much. It's part of nature and I knew at some point that my body would alter. An occasional hot flash might be annoying but since I know what's causing it—and that it's not forever—I can deal with it. What I'm here for is something else. Joe and I have been married for eighteen years, and I've always been the sexual aggressor. It works for us, and we like it. However, in the last few months I've become passive, and both my husband and I are wondering what to do. We both want what we had to continue."

I told Margaret that there was a great possibility that her testosterone levels were lower than usual, given her age and menopausal status. Her blood tests bore this out: Her levels were deficient. In order to boost her estrogen levels at the same time, I prescribed Estratest H.S. (for Half Strength), a low-dose combination of both estrogen and testosterone.

After a month, Margaret called with good news.

"It's working. My sex drive is back and my husband is delighted. As am I."

Although it's thought of as an exclusively male hormone, testosterone is not limited to men. Women produce small amounts in their ovaries, adrenal glands, and fat cells. While there are wide variances in levels, a woman, generally speaking, has about 5 to 10 percent as much testosterone as a man.

The complete role of testosterone in women still isn't known. What is understood is that, for some postmenopausal women, a decline in testosterone can cause thinning pubic hair, declining libido, a reduction in overall muscle mass, and loss of memory.

If a woman's blood test reveals that her testosterone levels are low—below the 20-to-60 ng/dl norm—*I prescribe Estratest H.S. This is a combination of .625 mg of estrogen and 1.25 mg of methyltestosterone, a synthetic hormone, in a single pill.* While this standard dosage works well for most people, some patients have achieved satisfaction with as little as one-quarter or one-half of this amount. However, for postmenopausal women with normal testosterone levels, the pill is not recommended; it produces no sexual boost.

Estratest H.S. raises sexual desire and prevents vaginal dryness. If this reduced dosage doesn't produce the desired effect, I recommend experimentation after consultation with your health-care provider.

Sometimes testosterone alone will impart the desired effect. I have had testosterone made up for some of my patients by a local compounding pharmacist into a 1-percent cream. This cream is rubbed into the arm or thigh every day to maintain desirable levels of testosterone. Other effective delivery routes for testosterone are oral and sublingual (or, under the tongue). Again, my compounding pharmacist has made up batches of .5 mg testosterone pills that my patients take daily. I like the sublingual route because the testosterone is dissolved in a matter of minutes under the tongue, where it is released directly into the bloodstream.

For now, as with testosterone supplementation for men, the long-term effects on women are unknown. On the one hand, some researchers believe that testosterone may prevent osteoporosis. On the other, it could reduce the beneficial effects that estrogen imparts on cholesterol levels.

While using testosterone, your physician should check your progress during scheduled visits, especially during the first few months of treatment. The dosage may have to be finely adjusted. My male patients are monitored regularly, and I check their prostate glands for signs of enlargement, a possible side effect of testosterone supplementation. Women are also examined systematically for any signs of virilization, marked by a deepened voice, acne, or facial hair. But at these low levels I have not witnessed any of these changes. Follow-up checks of testosterone blood levels may also be helpful in guiding therapy.

Nitroglycerine

Barry and Kate, both my patients for a number of years, arrived for their checkups with something very specific in mind.

"Barry and I have always had a fine sex life," Kate began. "But frankly, a little experimentation is in order. After fifteen years together, we think we're stable enough to try something new."

I recommended a special nitroglycerine ointment and instructed them on its use.

By the following Monday, Barry was on the phone. "The ointment worked—in minutes. It gave us an exciting boost and it's something we'll save for special occasions, like a good bottle of wine."

The Nitroglycerine Facts

An effective vasodilator of arteries and veins, nitroglycerine has traditionally been used to treat coronary artery disease, angina in particular. However, beneficial effects of nitroglycerine have also been felt in penile erectile tissue.

Once nitroglycerine is applied to the skin it's absorbed immediately into the bloodstream, causing blood vessels to widen. When applied directly to the penis, more blood flows into it, resulting in an erection.

I recommend a 2 percent nitroglycerine prescription ointment. It should be applied to a one-inch surface of the penis thirty to sixty minutes before intercourse. Remember: To effectively prevent the transmission of the drug to the sex partner, which will result in a headache, a man must use a condom. The ointment can also be applied to the perineal area, the space between the anus and the scrotum. If you choose this application, nitroglycerine will not be transmitted to the partner and a condom does not have to be worn.

Sensual Touch: The Vital Connection

Something we cannot live without, touch is something we crave as soon as we're born. Slow, sensual touch can do more to foster intimacy and love than all the sexual gymnastics put together. Nature intended it this way. Look at your fingertips: They're outfitted with fleshy pads at the tips that allow greater sensitivity and responsiveness to stimuli. Think about the things we touch—the head of a baby, a silk tie, the page of a book. We long for tactile sensation and actively seek it out. Skin is our largest organ and a sensory receptor of epic proportion.

If there is one drawback to the pleasures of touching it's this: It takes time. That means it requires respect, slowing down the pace of our lives in order to allow its effects to be fully felt and appreciated.

I recommend to my patients that they take the time to explore their partners in nonsexual ways. That way, they can:

- expand their interpersonal relationships
- find out how each partner likes to touch and be touched
- explore nonsexual patterns of offering pleasure without pressure to perform sexually
- provide feedback to the giver about what feels good and how he or she is able to do it
- increase oxytocin levels to help establish a strong bond between partners

The Oxytocin Bond

New research in the field of pharmacosexology is exploring the effects of certain hormones on the heightening of initial sexual feelings, stimulation to seek sex, and sexual pleasure itself. Most of us are familiar with endorphins, those elusive feel-good substances that drift through the bloodstream and produce the so-called runner's high. Released during the course of aerobic exercise, endorphins continue to affect one's mood long after the workout is over.

But when it comes to sexuality, oxytocin is the hormone that is beginning to be noticed and studied. For many years, oxytocin was regarded by researchers as a secondary hormone secreted by the pituitary gland. Its function was thought to be limited to female reproduction. Oxytocin is pivotal in relaxing the uterus so that birth can take place. After that, it contributes to the process that allows postpartum lactation to begin.

About ten years ago, researchers began to investigate oxytocin's other effects on laboratory animals. More recently, oxytocin has been found in a number of sites previously unknown, including the brainstem, spinal cord, and limbic system. In animal studies using virgin female rats, oxytocin introduced into their brains produced startling results: The rodents became total maternal role models, responding to the needs of offspring that didn't belong to them.

Subsequent studies focused on the successful mating habits of rats when oxytocin was introduced. Research was also done on the elevated levels of oxytocin found in the bloodstream of animals and humans (both male and female) after mating.

It is eminently clear that oxytocin, by promoting loving feelings between partners, is intricately involved in the process of intimacy, romance, and mating. It may even be partially responsible for the rhythmic spasms felt during orgasm.

Stored in the pituitary gland, oxytocin is easy to access: Touching, holding, caressing—all lead to its release, which in turn accentuates feelings of warmth and love toward the receiving person. And the best thing about oxytocin is that we can trigger its release on demand. I encourage all my patients to hold and hug as much as possible. This behavior evokes wonderful health benefits by promoting sensual communication, maximizing sexual arousal, and paving the way for optimal fulfillment for both people involved.

Note: The release of oxytocin can also be stimulated by using angelica, an herbal root. Native American women have long used this herb as an aid in the birthing process. Brewing tea is simple: Put a teaspoonful of the cut root in a cup of water and bring it to a boil. Let it stand for fifteen minutes before drinking. One cup three times daily will promote the release of oxytocin.

The Role of Exercise

"I knew that having that stupid cast on my leg would slow me down," complained Andrew, a fifty-one-year-old insurance company executive, "but I didn't think its effects would last after I took it off."

When I asked him if he was referring to the aftereffects of reconstructive surgery on a snapped Achilles' tendon, the result of sprinting to first base in a summer softball game, he nodded. I pointed out that once he started weight training and running, slowly, to build up stamina, the powerful outline of muscles on his legs would return. He was going to make a full recovery. But something else was bothering him as well.

"Actually, I've slowed down a lot in the bedroom, too," he admitted. "Before the accident things were great between Sue and me. We had sex several times a week, and we both looked forward to it. It's been a very important aspect of our marriage—and we've been together over twenty years. But in the last few weeks it has all seemed to change. Okay—since the surgery I've put on ten pounds. That I can take care of; but I'm a lot more concerned that somewhere along the way my sex drive snapped, too."

When he listened to my diagnosis—no exercise in almost two months was sure to reduce a sex drive—his face brightened considerably.

Regular exercise equals better sex, I told him. There's a definite connection between being physically active and sustaining an energetic sex life. And the converse is true as well: Stopping exercise can put the brakes on sexual drive. Andrew was prevented from performing his regular exercise routine and, therefore, his sexual performance suffered. But since he couldn't run at his usual pace yet, I suggested he take up another exercise in the interim. Swimming was a natural choice, along with riding a bicycle. And while these exertions wouldn't help him prepare for a New York City Marathon run, they would certainly aid in revving up his sex life.

Andrew took my advice. Three weeks later, after swimming laps at the local YMCA pool and pedaling on a stationary bicycle afterward several times a week, he was relieved. "You were right," he reported. "I may not be back to competitive speed on the track, but I'm where I want to be with Sue. The best thing about your 'prescription' is that I'm using my body to heal myself."

The Exercise/Sex Connection

As many of you will readily attest, exercise is one of the most effective sex enhancers. A regular program can quickly translate into an improved sex life; research in this area emphatically points out that those people who exercise regularly tend to be more active sexually as well. I strongly believe in the power of body movement to spur a sluggish libido, and I always encourage men and women to exercise on a regular, if not daily, basis. Recent studies concur:

• Men who participated in a nine-month basic running program were found to increase their frequency of sexual intercourse significantly. Beginning at an average of having sex seven times a month at the start of the program, they were averaging twelve times a month by its end.

• Women ranging in age from twenty-two to sixty years of age reported a 30 percent jump in their frequency of sexual activity after three months in an aerobics class.

• A study comparing the level of sexual activity found in groups of sedentary subjects with a coed group of swimmers, all over the age of twenty-five, who raced regularly throughout the year reinforces the connection between exercise and sex. Compared to their nonactive counterparts, the swimmers reported a much higher incidence of sexual intercourse.

Sex, of course, is not just a physical act. It's a finely tuned interaction of both mind and body. Therefore, it's difficult for researchers to assess the "quality" of sex quantitatively. While increased sexual frequency doesn't guarantee better sex, at least one study, involving nonexercising California men, has found this to be true.

Over a nine-month period, researchers put seventy-eight of their subjects on a program consisting of calisthenics, slow jogging, and stationary bicycle riding. They performed these functions three times a week for a period of an hour. By contrast, a control group of seventeen sedentary men were monitored as they exercised moderately, walking at a leisurely pace for an hour, four times a week.

At the end of the study, the sexual habits of the walking group showed no significant changes. However, a look at the diaries kept by the more active group revealed an entirely different story. Their personal notations revealed that, as the workout program progressed, so did their sex lives. All noted more deep kissing, more sex on a regular basis, and more frequent and satisfying orgasms.

Although exercise can be a powerful sex enhancer, the "whys" of just how it improves sex are not yet fully understood. At the most basic level, we know that regular exercise improves overall physical fitness, and that sexual functioning is an important part of that condition. We also know that regular exercise:

- positively affects brain wave activity, making you feel more energized
- raises body temperature, duplicating one of the main reactions associated with arousal
- increases stamina, preventing or delaying fatigue during sex
- builds muscle strength, helping to heighten sexual response—orgasm requires considerable muscle activity
- augments testosterone levels in both men and women, leading to increased libido
- decreases the percentage of body fat, which in turn can positively alter personal attitudes regarding sex
- improves cardiovascular function, which causes vasocongestion, or increased blood supply to the penis during intercourse, thereby helping to achieve and maintain an erection

Improving Vasocongestion

One of the most consequential physical responses triggered by sexual excitement, vasocongestion is the increased flow of blood to the genitals. In men, as noted above, vasocongestion leads to an erection, while in women, the uterus, clitoris, and labia become engorged with blood, prompting the lubrication of genital tissues with a vaginal secretion. Both sexes experience an increase in heart rate, respiration, and blood pressure as well.

The degree and frequency of vasocongestion depend on healthy, unobstructed blood vessels (the heart isn't the only organ affected adversely by clogged arteries). Blockages or narrowing of arteries in the penis will limit blood flow, resulting in difficulties in achieving and maintaining an erection.

Because these blood vessels tend to clog earlier than those of the heart, impotence due to artery damage can also be an early indicator of heart trouble. However, regular aerobic exercise, such as walking briskly, running, or swimming laps all for twenty minutes or more, has several beneficial health effects. Not only will it improve the efficiency of your cardiovascular system, but it can help promote vasocongestion and protect against impotence problems.

Sex-Enhancing Exercises

Since most of the body's major muscles are utilized during sex, exercise with any kind of resistance equipment to develop muscle strength and endurance can quickly translate into improved sexual performance. Particular attention should be paid to the large muscles of the abdomen, hips, and thighs; sexual activity makes active use of all of them.

However, there is a set of muscles that get little, if any, attention on a regular basis: the pubococcygeus (PC) muscles, the set of muscles and ligaments that supports the bladder and is located around the genitals in the region between the legs defined as the pelvic floor. Exercising and strengthening them can go a long way toward greatly enhancing your sex life. These are the same muscles you squeeze to stop the flow of urine. To locate your PC muscles and test their current force, the next time you have to urinate, tense the muscles, stopping and restarting the urine stream. If you can do this easily, your PC muscles are probably well-toned. If the flow continues despite your efforts, then these muscles are probably in need of a workout. If this is the case, check out Kegels, exercises for strengthening the pelvic diaphragm and pubic area that were developed by a gynecologist, and Callanetics, a popular calisthenic exercise program. Both develop this muscle area.

An Important Caveat About Exercise

I would never suggest that exercise is bad. However, under certain circumstances it can adversely affect your sex life. I have known patients who have used exercise as a substitute for sex, and those who worked out so hard that they were good for nothing, much less a satisfying sexual encounter, afterward. For instance, if you are running a marathon and know you will be exhausted, don't have a lot of expectations for a night of sexual romping. If you're tired after work and then work out, you may find yourself further depleted of energy. Listen to your body and respect what it tells you. If you do, you won't be disappointed.

Effects of Drugs on Sexual Function

Many common prescription drugs can adversely affect sexual functioning in both men and women. Desire, arousal, and orgasm, as well as erection and ejaculation, are all susceptible. There are also drugs (alcohol, for example) that encourage arousal but inhibit erection and orgasm. However, there is such a wide range of drugs now available that a knowledgeable physician can usually remedy the situation by substituting one drug for another to eliminate or reduce sexual side effects.

Unwanted sexual side effects are caused most often by drugs prescribed for hypertension (high blood pressure)

SUMMARY OF NEW APHRODISIACS AND RECOMMENDATIONS

Source	What It Does	Daily Recommendations
L-arginine	Essential amino acid affects blood flow, triggering nitric oxide, which causes erection	Supplements available in health food stores; 2 g in the evening (if herpes is a factor, add 1 gram of lysine)
Yohimbe	Active chemical helps erectile problems, increases sex drive in men; no current studies on effects on women	Synthetic or herbal form 5.4 mg tablets taken three times a day
Deprenyl	Prescription drug stimulates dopamine, increasing libido and enjoyment	Age 40–50: 5 mg three times a week; age 50–60: 5 mg four times a week; age 60–70: 5 mg daily
Trazodone	Antidepressant stimulates muscle relaxation, leading to erection in men; prescribed for women who are mildly depressed and fatigued	Begin with 50 mg daily; dosage changes based on physician's recommendation
Testosterone	Hormone that regulates sex drive in men and women; used to improve libido	For men: physician's prescription injection followed by 2.5 mg transdermal patches; for women: Estratest H.S. .625 mg of estrogen and 1.25 mg of methyltestosterone (¼ to ½ dosage may be ideal); .5 mg sublingual testosterone tablet or 1% topical cream
Nitroglycerine	Vasodilator leads to erection	Apply prescription 2% nitroglycerine ointment to the penis 30 to 60 minutes before intercourse; condom must be used

Source	What It Does	Daily Recommendations
Sensual touch	Stimulates oxytocin, which is linked to physical sensation and intimacy; sharpens dopamine's effect on sexual pleasure, enhances orgasm	Foreplay, including sufficient caressing and touching; one cup of angelica tea three times a day can increase oxytocin levels
Exercise	Increases blood flow to the genitals, affecting brain wave activity, increasing energy, sex drive, and frequency	20 to 40 minutes of continuous physical activity daily

and psychiatric conditions. While not all men and women using these drugs experience these problems, you should watch for any of the following when taking prescription medications:

- depressed libido
- arousal difficulties
- breast enlargement in men
- reduced sexual frequency
- impaired vaginal lubrication
- inability to ejaculate
- diminished orgasms
- impotence

Note: Testosterone levels can be lowered and sperm production impaired by certain drugs. Tests can be performed to see if you are experiencing these particular side effects.

What You Can Do

The major obstacle to identifying and solving sexual problems stemming from prescription drugs is, sadly, a general lack of awareness on the part of the person taking the medication. Many people ignore what could be the obvious culprit, instead, blaming marital woes, work-related stress, or aging.

The first step toward alleviating sexual difficulty is to determine whether it could be related to any prescription medication. If the problem began shortly after the course of medication started, the drug probably is responsible for the sexual difficulty at hand. In that case, there are options to consider:

• If the problem is only mildly annoying, or if the drug must be taken for only a short period of time, it may be reasonable to continue the full course of medication. If, however, the medical problem arises in the future, ask your doctor for an alternate drug.

• If the medication is for a chronic condition such as hypertension or depression, and your normal sex life has been negatively affected by it, your doctor can experiment with lower doses, or with other medications or combinations of drugs.

Whatever you do, *don't reduce the dosage on your own or stop taking a medication.* This could prove to be dangerous to your health. Always discuss your problem and attainable choices with your physician. By keeping communication open and clear between you and your doctor, you can work together to change or adjust your medication. The goal is to ensure that your health is maintained and your sexual functioning preserved.

Drugs That Affect Sexual Function

The following medications may have a detrimental effect on sexual function in men and women. If you are taking any of the following drugs and experiencing unwanted side effects, call your doctor and ask for a substitute.

Antiparasite: Flagyl

Antacid: Bentyl, Combid, and Tagamet

Antidepression/antianxiety: Anafranil, Asapin, Asendin, Elavil, Endep, Ludiomil, Mellaril, Nardil, Navane, Norpramin, Pamelor, Parnate, Paxil, Prozac, Sinequan, Stelazine, Tofranil, Valium, Vivactyl, Zoloft

Antihypertension: Aldomet, Aldactone, Atenolol, Blocadren, Captopril,* Catapres, Diltiazem, Enalapril,* Inderal, Labetalol, Lasix, Lisinopril,* Lopressor, Nifedipine, Prazosin, Tenex, Terazosin, Verapamil

Appetite suppressants: Fastin, Ionamin, Tenuate

Cholesterol-lowerers: Atromid-S

Muscle relaxants: Flexeril

Saving the Libido from the Impact of Prozac

Louis, a forty-eight-year-old business executive, had been on the receiving end of a downsizing at his company. Seven months later, still out of work and despairing over his opportunities, he came to see me.

He was visibly depressed; he didn't shake my hand when he came into my office and never smiled. "I know it's normal to be 'down' when you lose your job. But this is different," he told me. "I feel apathetic, unconnected. I don't feel any joy at all, not with my wife, my daughters, anything. For the first time in my life I think I'm depressed."

After further discussions, it became apparent that Louis was in fact accurate in his assessment. We discussed the various treatments available and I explained which antidepressant medications would offer him the most effective and quickest response. We then agreed that Louis would try the antidepressant Prozac to raise his spirits.

A disabling illness thought to be caused by biochemical imbalances in the brain, depression is unfortunately very prevalent: Over four million Americans experience it every year. However, the good news is that it can be treated effectively with medication. Fluoxetine (Prozac), a drug in the selective serotonin re-uptake inhibitor (SSRI) class that

---

*Note: These drugs do not decrease libido at normal dosages.

was introduced in the late 1980s, has become quite popular in the treatment of mild to moderate forms of depression. Still, while they have proven to be effective in treating depression, some antidepressants, and the SSRIs in particular, can produce troublesome side effects in up to one-third of the men and women who take them. Common sexual problems can include diminished libido, change in arousal sensitivity, and difficulties in reaching orgasm. Some people develop these side effects within days. In Louis's case it took longer.

After three months on Prozac, Louis informed me that he was feeling much better, brighter, able to enjoy life again. He had found a new job closer to home, thereby eliminating the long commute he had once faced. He could now spend more time with his family. Unfortunately, he had another report to make as well.

"It's pretty ironic to say I feel great when my sex life has evaporated," he told me. "I have no trouble getting an erection. But it takes so long to reach orgasm—if it happens at all. It looks to me like I have a lousy choice: Stop taking the medication, feel lousy, and not be interested in sex, or take it and give up on sex. Needless to say, I certainly don't want to do that."

I told Louis that before 1996 reports of sexual problems caused by antidepressants had been anecdotal, just passing from patient to physician. That year, however, two double-blind studies, in which neither patients nor physicians knew who was using which drug, finally confirmed that SSRIs are, in fact, responsible for sexual problems. Fortunately, the studies also uncovered a possible solution. A medication called nefazodone (Serzone), which has some SSRI properties, is less likely than other drugs to trigger sexual dysfunction. The two studies found that while Serzone and Zoloft, a popular SSRI similar to Prozac and Paxil, both worked well in combating depression, those men and women who had been taking Serzone had fewer sexual difficulties.

I switched Louis to Serzone, and two weeks later was happy to hear from him that his unwanted side effect had disappeared.

Another of my patients, a thirty-two-year-old woman

taking Prozac for depression, complained of a new difficulty in reaching orgasm which, in turn, affected her desire for sex. Since her depression was under control, she asked if she could go off it on weekends. Because Prozac's effects are long-lasting, I agreed. The "drug-free weekend" brought about a return of desire.

While Prozac certainly has helped many patients overcome depression, most of my older patients still use the earlier tricyclic antidepressants, such as Elavil (amitriptyline) and Tofranil (imipramine). Unfortunately, these drugs can have an anticholinergic effect—that is, dampen sexual drive and desire. I have had great success with these patients by prescribing a cholinergic drug, bethanechol chloride. Taken in 12.5 to 25 mg doses daily in conjunction with antidepressant medication, this drug dramatically reverses orgasmic dysfunction.

Another medication I have also found to be very helpful in restoring sexual energy while combating depression is Wellbutrin (bupropion). Like Serzone, Wellbutrin does not suppress a patient's sex drive nor does it interfere with sexual performance. However, unlike Serzone, which affects the brain's serotonin neurotransmitters, Wellbutrin is thought to enhance the activity of dopamine receptors in the brain. The beauty of this prescription drug is that it helps restore the sex drive of a patient, in some instances actually acting as a quasi-aphrodisiac. I have had several patients report that their libido increased significantly while they were using the medication.

Birth Control Pills and Sex Drive

Jane, a thirty-four-year-old artist, called me a couple of months after she began to take a new birth control pill.

"Why were you holding back information from me?" she asked. "Those new pills have changed my life."

For years, Jane had been taking Orthonovum 1/35. This pill produces the same level of progestin, an important hormonal component, throughout her twenty-one-day cycle. Progestin, or progesterone, stimulates the lining of the uterus in preparation for pregnancy. It peaks during the second half of the menstrual cycle. However, at her sister's suggestion, Jane had asked me to switch her to Orthonovum 7/7/7, a triphasic pill that varies the level of progestin during the monthly cycle.

"After just a week on the new pills my sexual desire hit levels I didn't know existed," she exclaimed. "My boyfriend actually said that he thought I'd turned into a nymphomaniac. My orgasms are much more intense and powerful. And I find myself fantasizing about sex on a daily basis."

I had to confess to her that I had not known that a birth control pill could actually enhance sexuality. Jane then admitted that her sister had experienced similar results, prompting her to try it.

My interest piqued, I did some investigation of my own. I found research done at San Francisco State University which strongly suggested that triphasic birth control pills boosted both libido and sexual satisfaction. In this study, Dr. Norma McCoy questioned 364 sexually active women between the ages of eighteen and twenty-six, less than half of whom used birth control pills. The seventy-three women who used the triphasic drug reported four distinct findings. They had increased sexual interest, number of sexual fantasies, arousal during sex, and satisfaction from intercourse.

To date, no one is certain why triphasic birth control pills trigger increased sexual interest and activity. Dr. McCoy has speculated that it could be due to the fact that triphasic pills delay the suppression of luteinizing hormone, which controls the production of other sex hormones.

If you're not satisfied with your current birth control pills, or find that they've diminished your libido, speak with your physician about switching medications.

Sex and Heart Attack

We've all heard stories about famous people—usually men—suffering a fatal heart attack while in the midst of a passionate sexual encounter. What are the real odds of this happening to you? Infinitesimally small.

Sexual activity is responsible for only about 1 percent of all heart attacks, with an estimated seven out of ten deaths occurring during an extramarital affair. Still, the odds of having a heart attack during sex are very slim. In fact, getting out of bed in the morning—a time when blood is more likely to form clots that can trigger a heart attack—is much riskier. Currently it accounts for 10 percent of all heart attacks.

According to research conducted by heart specialist James E. Muller, M.D., a physician at Deaconess Hospital in Boston, your risk of heart attack before sex is one in a million. Your chances do begin to rise during a sexual encounter, but they only move up a notch to two in a million both during and after intercourse.

Unfortunately, heart disease is quite common and a very serious health matter. Some of my patients between the ages of forty and fifty have already suffered their first heart attacks. Even so, heart disease doesn't mean that sexual intimacy has to end. Studies of men and women recovering from heart attacks have shown that sex is an activity avoided by both sexes out of misguided fear. They believe that sex is hazardous to their health, that pleasure will quickly and inevitably translate into pain when the exertion of intercourse induces another cardiac episode.

There is no question that heart disease is a serious health concern. But having had a heart attack is not a reason to scare yourself into celibacy. Sadly, it's estimated that as many as 70 percent of men who have had heart attacks find reasons to avoid sex afterward. They doubt the safety of having sex, even after having waited the recommended four to six weeks before resuming intimate relations.

The good news is that recent research by Dr. Muller has determined that sexual intercourse is highly unlikely to cause another attack. His 1996 study, which involved 1,774 patients who had suffered a heart attack, revealed that they temporarily raised their risk of another attack from ten in a million to twenty in a million. However, since the starting dangers are so low to begin with, even doubling them is a low-risk venture.

Stress and the Sexual Urge

Work and financial demands, concerns over raising children and taking care of elderly parents—all these pressures, and many more, have pushed sex far from the center stage of many couples' lives. Not surprisingly, it has become a major source of conflict between them instead of a shared source of joy. I've heard the following complaints far too often:

"We put so much time into our jobs, trying to keep up the mortgage payments and college tuition for our kids, that there's barely any energy—which means much less time for sex."

"When we do make love it often seems hurried, unsatisfactory. I hate to admit it, but I think we're just too tired to enjoy sex anymore."

"I just don't have time for sex."

"He's not interested like I am."

"She's lost interest in me."

"His sex drive is low."

"Her sex drive is nonexistent."

In most of these cases the problems aren't physical—all the equipment needed is in fine working order. Rather, its roots are psychological, and linked directly to the stresses of everyday life.

Stress and Sexual Arousal

Sexual arousal, which includes the surging of blood, increased heart rate, nipple and penile erection, and deep breathing, depends in great part on a number of hormones to play their specific roles. These hormones are chemical messengers that spark specific reactions in the body.

For instance, there is the role of adrenaline, a hormone that can adversely affect libido. Whenever you're under stress, no matter the source, adrenaline starts to course through your veins, directing blood flow to major muscles—and away from the genitals—preparing you for a "fight or flight" response. This reaction is a genetic inheritance from our ancient ancestors, who experienced a similar sensation whenever they came face to face with a charging beast.

If the stress is removed, then some normalcy returns. However, if you're under constant stress all day, something I call a state of "distress"—whether it be from concern about job performance, a fight with a spouse or co-worker, or money problems—sex is anything but a priority.

Then there is the vital sex hormone testosterone, which also falls victim to the effects of stress on men and women. Literally our "sex fuel" (all it takes is a little to turn on our sex drive), testosterone is extremely sensitive to stress. Even a small amount of outside pressure can shut off our sexual impulses. Studies with soldiers preparing to head into battle have proved it. Testosterone levels plummeted when the soldiers were facing their enemy, only to rise again after their return to safety.

Sex: The Prescription for Defusing Stress

Surprisingly, sex is one of the best stress relievers going. The only problem many people have is finding enough time to give it the respect it deserves. For stressed-out partners, my immediate recommendation is for a romantic interlude. Determined, of course, by the individual tastes of the people involved, that can mean whatever suits—a peaceful walk in a park, a late-afternoon lunch in a quiet restaurant, enacting an erotic fantasy, a ride in the country—followed by private time at home, with the telephone off the hook. Or it can be a much-needed weekend getaway, far from children and job pressures. Basically, it's a chance to slow down, recharge sexual batteries, and intimately rediscover each other. Remember, romance isn't something reserved only for anniversaries and birthdays; it's a wonderful part of life that should be embraced as much as possible.

A healthy sexual life is built on attention, to yourself and your partner. It has to be nurtured, and will repay you both in innumerable, satisfying ways.

4

The New Image Revolution

Looking as good as you possibly can, no matter what your age, is no longer a dream: The tools that can make it happen are available right now. We all know that when we look good we feel good, suffused with confidence, energized, and positive. I believe that presenting an attractive exterior mirrors a healthy attitude about who we are and how well we are taking care of ourselves. It's obvious: If you don't feel well you can't look great; it's also true that an outward appearance that doesn't match the image you'd like to project may make you feel less than terrific.

In our society, where the physical attributes of youth continue to be idealized, a toned, smooth body and wrinkle-free face is an ideal for anyone in the competitive workplace. The idea is that if you look young you will project a fresh, appealing demeanor that will be felt at work and in your personal life.

My patients have been very vocal about their need to maintain and enhance their appearance, and I am delighted to tell them that brand-new technologies are making their aims not only attainable but longer lasting and more effective than ever before. Today, there is a whole new world of physical enrichment available, based on science, research, and the very real needs of people who are embracing its possibilities. We can now:

- reduce cellulite and recontour the body without surgery
- erase age spots, lines, and wrinkles from faces in an out-patient procedure
- repair and protect sun-damaged skin using natural substances

Cellulite: What It Is

Cellulite is the physical trait that annoys my female patients above all others. Although it's not a health problem, cellulite is a significant cosmetic one that has, in the past, managed to evade erasure.

Ask most physicians what cellulite is and they'll tell you that there is no such thing. Cellulite, they say, is a made-up word that means fat, and all body fat is the same. I disagree: While all body fat may be the same, where it is located on the body, and what it does to skin appearance, especially for women, is a different matter altogether.

The appearance of cellulite changes with age, and can be categorized into three distinct stages. These specific phases are classified as:

Stage 1: The skin surface is smooth while standing or lying down. However, when the skin on the thighs or buttocks is gently pinched, a dimpling of the skin—the so-called mattress phenomenon—can be seen. This is common for all women.

Stage 2: When lying down, the skin surface is smooth. Upon standing the cellulite on hips, thighs, and buttocks is very visible. This is common for women over thirty-five or those who are obese.

Stage 3: The "mattress phenomenon" is visible when standing and lying down. This is quite common for women who put on extra weight, as well as those past menopause.

Out of reproductive necessity, women have more fat then men. While a typically fit male has 18 percent body fat, a fit woman has closer to 25 percent. And a woman's body fat is held in place differently as well. Tiny connective tissue strands called septa hold fat cells together, linking the fat to the skin layer above and the muscle below to form a protective cushion.

In males, the septa follow a neat crisscrossed, thatched pattern, imparting skin tone with a consistently smooth appearance. In women, the septa are thought to be arranged in vertical rows; however, there are new data that suggest a crisscross pattern as well. When fat cells expand and increase in size—and they can swell two hundred to three hundred times their normal size due to weight gain—or when they lose their elasticity and shrink with age, lymphatic circulation between fat cells slows down, resulting in a circulatory and water-retention problem. This combination of swollen fat cells and shortened septa pulls down on the skin, causing it to contract.

The result is cellulite, those lumpy areas on hips, thighs, and buttocks that bother women enormously, provoking them to find ways to rid themselves of it.

Endermologie: The Cellulite Solution

When Elaine came for her yearly checkup, she had a single complaint. At forty-six, this very stylish party planner looked terrific. All except for one thing.

"I can't stand this cellulite. I've had it since I was a teenager and thirty years is enough. I thought that losing all that weight would have eliminated this awful 'fat.' But it's still here, and I'm still not wearing bathing suits at the beach."

Four years before, Elaine had lost a significant amount of weight. Using my *Thinner at Last* program that combines the use of two weight-loss medications, fenfluramine and phentermine, she took ninety pounds off her five-foot five-inch frame in eighteen months. She also revamped her eating habits and started to exercise regularly, toning and shaping her body as much as she could. Her goal had been to restore herself to her prepregnancy form and indeed, she had succeeded well beyond that expectation. In fact, she was in better shape than she had been sixteen years before.

But for all of her exercising—she ran every morning before work and lifted weights twice a week—the cellulite remained. Sporting a trim and muscled body, she felt that her remaining physical flaw was her thighs, which refused to be diminished, much less reshaped.

"I'm doing everything I can. Why won't it go away?" she asked, gripping a thigh in each hand. "It was actually easier to live with when I was so overweight because then my whole body was out of shape. But now that the rest of me looks better there's an even greater contrast between the way I look above and below my waist."

I was delighted to inform Elaine of a new, proven, noninvasive treatment for cellulite that is now available in the United States. Not a surgical procedure, Endermologie is a remarkable invention that has been in use in France for the past five years.

I explained that the procedure was very simple. In essence, a patented machine is used that can actually deeply massage the offending areas into something the mirror has not shown you before. Endermologie is a patented technique, which combines powerful suction and motorized roller heads, providing deep benefits to soft tissue by promoting the drainage of fluids and stretching the septa, or connective tissues. Circulation is increased, the removal of intercellular waste is speeded up, and connective tissues are softened, their elasticity restored. Over time, irregular contours are smoothed and the appearance of cellulite is decreased. When combined with regular exercise and low-fat eating, the results I have seen on my patients are very impressive.

When I showed Elaine photographic proof of success (all pictures were of bodies only; no faces are ever recorded) she was ready and willing to try Endermologie.

"Sign me up," she ordered. "I've been waiting my whole life for something like this."

The Endermologie Effects

For Elaine, *my recommendation, to achieve maximal results, was to have twice-weekly, thirty-five-minute sessions for seven weeks.* I explained that the sessions are vigorous, and each one needs to be spaced at least forty-eight hours apart. That way, the removal of waste products is facilitated, and the body has time to rest.

Changes in skin tone, cellulite reduction, and body contouring often become apparent by the sixth or seventh session. Some of the first things noticed are:

- diminished or erased cellulite lumps and bulges
- smoother skin: rough patches are evened out, their texture made tauter and firmer
- better-fitting clothing

The Endermologie Session

I introduced Elaine to Denise, the therapist who works with many of my patients. She explained to Elaine that she would first be photographed, so that her progress could be documented. After being properly positioned, Elaine was photographed nine times to show front, rear, and profile views. She would be photographed again, in the same positions, after the ninth and fourteenth sessions so that changes in body contour and skin quality could be monitored accurately.

Next, she would pull on a pair of sheer, queen-size pantyhose specially designed for this procedure, over her underwear, up to her chest. This is a sanitary precaution which prevents body hair and oils, as well as dead skin cells, from clogging the machine. Also, it acts as a micro-thin barrier between the treatment head and the skin, helping the tool to glide easily over the body.

Denise showed Elaine the rollerheads of the machine, pointing out that the power settings can be switched from a very mild number one to a very powerful number ten. Usually, as treatments progress the power is increased, since the person receiving Endermologie is more relaxed and can tolerate more as time goes on. She told Elaine to let her know if she felt any discomfort, no matter what the setting was; everyone has different sensitivities in various parts of the body. The goal of the treatment was to manipulate connective tissue as well as increase venous and lymphatic circulation. It would also make her skin more supple, diminish muscular tension, and help to reshape her lower body.

Instructing her to lie facedown on a massage table, Denise began the session. She rolled the machine over Elaine's hips, thighs, and buttocks in various motions, pulling the fat under the skin to stimulate waste removal. Then she worked on sculpting and contouring the problem areas. Afterwards, she asked Elaine to roll over onto her back so that she could work on the front of her legs as well as inner thighs, stomach, and abdomen. Finally, she worked on her underarms as well. When Elaine's skin was rosy, it meant that circulation was increasing.

After the session, Denise told Elaine not to be surprised if, the following day, she noticed some bruising, which would quickly disappear. And she also reminded her, as she would at every other session, to make sure she drank a prescribed amount of water every day and exercised.

After the seven-week program Elaine came to see me. "Over the phone I can't possibly describe how well Endermologie worked," she said. "I just have to show you." I absolutely agreed; the change was dramatic. Elaine's bumps and bulges were significantly smaller, her skin considerably smoother, and the satisfied glow on her face spoke more vividly than anything else.

Endermologie: How It Works

I first heard about this amazing procedure from a patient who works as a massage therapist. She told me of a client who had returned from a yearlong stay in France. Immediately noticeable were her legs: Formerly streaked with cellulite, the woman's limbs were much smoother, the cellulite all but gone. While she had been in Paris, the woman told her, she had received Endermologie treatments from a local physician.

Not only was I intrigued by the story, I was incredulous

as well. Like most doctors, I was convinced that there was no effective treatment for cellulite. But my opinion was changed when I visited the Endermologie American headquarters, located in Fort Lauderdale, Florida. There, I met at length with their research team and had a chance to speak with therapists who had worked on both men and women in this country.

In addition, I reviewed hundreds of "before" and "after" photos of clients, which offered proof of the machine's amazing therapeutic properties. I came away convinced that the cellulite solution that has eluded us for so long was finally at hand.

Just how the machine accomplishes this is as mysterious as the process by which some blood pressure medications do their job. All we know is that the proof is clearly, empirically there. Currently, an MRI study is being done to determine exactly how the treatments work.

Nathalie Guitay, daughter of the machine's inventor and president of the American company, explained the Endermologie process to me. "This is not a miracle machine, but rather a mechanical device that helps the body to function normally. We think that it helps to stop intercellular swelling by allowing the body to give off waste products and free fatty acids—the way it is supposed to do. When this happens, fat cells shrink, the septa become more stimulated and nourished. This allows them to stretch to their full length, which is what makes the dimpled skin of cellulite disappear."

The Discovery of the Process

Endermologie, like cellulite, is a French word that won't be found in a medical dictionary. Created by Louis Paul Guitay, the term means "through the derm," or the skin, referring to the incredible ability of his Endermologie machine to work noninvasively.

Guitay, a forty-five-year-old engineer and inventor, discovered the process by chance. The victim of a car accident, he was left with a seriously injured left arm whose skin, from shoulder to wrist, was scraped off. His recuperation was slow, and he felt constant pain. But he found that as soon as physical therapy using massage was begun, mobility began to be restored to his arm, and his pain was lessened. But this was not surprising. The therapeutic effect of massage is hardly new; it is one of the oldest known body therapies. The rubbing, kneading, and pressing with various degrees of pressure that constitute massage help to improve circulation in the skin and muscles. Additionally, the pressure applied during massage seems to relieve pain, at least temporarily.

For Guitay, the weeks of twice-daily rehabilitation with his physical therapist were trying, but the deep massage strokes, as well as the application of friction to the skin's surface, began to show results that went beyond what he had expected. After a while, he noticed that his late-afternoon massage was not so intense as the one given in the morning and not so effective. He concluded that his physical therapist was tired by the end of the day, and therefore just couldn't give him as powerful a manipulation. The strength and depth of the massage were what appeared to make all the difference.

For Guitay, the solution to the promise of a consistently forceful massage every time was clear: A suction machine could do it. With such a device he could lift and manipulate scar tissue, as well as the underlying layers of nerve, muscle, and fat. He looked around his house and found his prototype: an electric vacuum cleaner.

Manipulating the nozzle over his arm in a lifting and rolling motion, Guitay worked on his arm for half an hour. The sensation was not unpleasant, and the results were very interesting: His skin tingled and glowed, the result of better circulation. Pleased with the outcome, he began twice-daily self-treatments.

After several weeks of observable improvement in the size and color of his scarred skin, Guitay was so convinced of the potential success of his method that he eliminated his sessions with the physical therapist. Continuing with his own therapy, he began to see the limitations of the vacuum cleaner. The suction head was just too small, which made his self-administered treatment sessions slow and tedious. This became a challenge he had to overcome. Inspired, he started to draw up ideas for a powerful machine that could suction and roll the skin with optimal results. His goal was twofold: to duplicate the work done by a therapist, as well as provide consistent and uniform results. His ultimate market would be people who were scarred or burned.

Guitay perfected his device until he was ready to form his own company to manufacture and distribute it. Used in the treatment of revitalizing scar tissue, his machine was taken up with enthusiasm by physical therapists throughout France.

However, during the course of treatment, many of the therapists noted that not only did the machine help improve blood supply to damaged skin and shrinking scars; it also improved the quality of healthy skin. Smoother, more pliable, and tauter, the skin was much better looking after treatments. Many women found that the cellulite on their thighs, hips, and buttocks was diminished. Some people even lost weight.

What was first a strictly therapeutic tool now had an enormous secondary application. Guitay began trials with women who were neither scarred nor burned to see if Endermologie could help reduce or eliminate cellulite. So promising were the results that his process has been embraced in his native country, and has finally crossed the ocean to the United States.

The Endermologie Facts

Access to the Endermologie machine, along with eyewitness observation, has impelled me to add this amazing process to my Vitality Medicine program. It's important to remember that Endermologie is not a "miracle" that will magically rid bodies of cellulite all by itself. Rather, it is a critical component in a simple, effective four-step program that I have developed. It includes these key elements:

1. a minimum of fourteen Endermologie treatments
2. a minimum of two liters of water drunk daily
3. proper nutrition
4. regular exercise

I have found that the people who are motivated to make changes in their lives and follow the four steps are the ones who achieve the best results. By adhering to this plan it's possible to bring about remarkable changes in all three cellulite stages. But those who first undergo Endermologie treatments before the age of thirty-five—and then continue them on a regular maintenance basis—will achieve the most beneficial results of all.

Endermologie: How to Begin

Once you have decided to try the treatment, your first step is to find a physician who understands the method. (For a physician in the New York, New Jersey, or Connecticut area, call 212-396-2516 for Endermologie centers in the New York tri-state area. For elsewhere in the United States, call 1-800-222-3911.) During your initial consultation, the doctor will take into consideration your unique physical characteristics to determine what is most effective for you. You will be asked to point out the specific areas you would like to see improved. Not only will this help the doctor understand your level of expectations; he or she will also be able to determine whether they can realistically be achieved. Exactly what can—and cannot—be done should be discussed between you and your doctor.

Those with more cellulite will see greater results, just as a person with more weight to lose will see a more profound outcome losing twenty pounds than the person who just needs to lose five.

At its best, Endermologie will improve both skin tone and reduce the level of cellulite, but it cannot promise perfection. Many of the women I have treated have experienced dramatic body contouring changes, but I must emphasize that results vary from patient to patient.

I have treated a number of obese patients—those thirty pounds over their ideal body weight—who wanted treatment for their cellulite. Endermologie has helped them. However, when obese patients are involved in a weight-loss program as well, there are numerous physiological changes going on and the treatment results are difficult to detect during this period. If the person still wants to undergo treatment while losing weight, I limit sessions to one per week, allowing more recovery time. The body needs to adapt to the metabolic shifting that takes place during weight loss.

What You Must Tell Your Doctor

Your doctor will need to know about any previous surgeries you may have had. Provide an accurate description about the effects of prior weight loss, as well as your exercise and eating regimens. Also, point out any scars or local skin discolorations so that they can be assessed to see if the treatment could affect them.

In all instances, I recommend that you discuss your medical status with your Endermologie treatment physician before starting a course of treatment. If any of the following apply to you, you must inform the physician.

• **Anticoagulant drugs.** Taking these medications may lead to easy bruising. Any person using an anticoagulant such as Coumadin is not a candidate. **Note:** If you take daily doses of aspirin you may experience bruising. Consult with your physician about a trial session.

• **Hernia.** Any rupture in the abdominal wall can be aggravated by the powerful suction force of the roller. Your physician must be made aware of previous hernias and hernia surgery.

• **Phlebitis.** This vein inflammation is usually associated with the formation of blood clots that can cause inflammation and obstruct blood flow. If you have this condition, you are not a candidate for treatment.

• **Pregnant women.** Because clinical evidence is lacking, any woman who is pregnant is not a candidate.

• **Pseudoatrophy.** Notify your doctor if you have received a recent cortisone injection. Several months after the shot an indentation, caused by it, may naturally appear on the skin.

• **Varicose veins.** All leg varicosities are avoided, with treatment administered around, but not directly on, damaged veins. Spider veins, however, can be improved because they react positively to increased circulation.

Why You Must Drink Two Liters of Water Daily

Not only is water crucial to life—about 60 percent of our body weight consists of this liquid—it plays an important role in the success of the Endermologie program. Every person who undergoes treatment is told to drink a minimum of two liters of water every day. Involved in every body process, from digestion to absorption, from circulation to elimination, water is a primary transporter of nutrients through the body. It is also the natural body cleanser that carries away waste products trapped by swollen cells.

Those practitioners who have had the most experience with Endermologie have found that increasing daily fluid intake ultimately gives the best results. When you have a session of Endermologie, you are hastening one of the waste elimination processes that your body performs daily. Drinking sufficient quantities of water is the most efficient way to carry eliminated impurities out of the body.

Remember that we are constantly losing water as a by-product of living. Breathing, perspiration, and elimination deplete the system of water throughout the day. You need to replenish the supply with at least two liters daily. Spread throughout the course of a day, this is a very manageable quantity to drink.

Many of my patients tell me that they reach the two-liter requirement by adding in all the coffee, tea, and soda they drink. Granted, these beverages are water-based, but since they also contain caffeine, a major dehydrating agent, their usefulness in fulfilling water requirements is limited. If you drink any of these beverages regularly, you can, however, count each cup as a half cup toward your overall water goal.

Beer, wine, and alcohol (which are also significant dehydrating agents) all prompt the kidneys to excrete more urine. None of these beverages can be counted in your two-liter water requirement. In fact, for every alcoholic drink taken, you will need to have one extra glass of water.

If you've lost count of just how much water you've had on a particular day, there's an easy way to check. If your urine is either pale yellow or clear, you're sufficiently hydrated.

Drinking water is particularly important when you exercise. It helps your cells absorb minerals, vitamins, amino acids, and glucose. It also rids the body of excess heat, cooling the body by producing sweat. With too little fluid your body simply won't be able to perform these functions effectively.

Why You Must Eat Properly

Anticellulite diets are a myth. When calories are restricted, weight is lost all over the body, not in specifically targeted areas. However, a sensible weight-loss program, in combination with exercise, which tones and tightens, will help improve the appearance of your skin. (I will discuss exercise at length in Chapter 7.)

The facts about weight loss are very basic:

1. How much you eat is the most consequential variable affecting weight.

2. Exercise is the other critical factor. To lose weight you must decrease the number of calories taken in and increase the amount of energy expended.

I offer my patients a number of nutritional options; each stresses a balanced approach to eating. We never discuss diets; instead, my patients and I focus on being "food aware." Food awareness is the opposite of dieting, because it relies on the individual to make informed choices and decisions throughout his or her day concerning what foods to eat, and portion size.

Maintaining consistent energy and vigor, planning rather than being coerced to eat something not wanted, and controlling health and healing through proper nutrition, are the goals and rewards of being "food aware." The cornerstone of being a food-aware eater is a low-fat, low-calorie regimen. The goal is to keep daily fat intake at no more than 30 percent of calories eaten; 20 percent is even better.

Questions and Answers About Endermologie

My patients always have questions about new treatments, and Endermologie is no exception. Here are the most often asked queries, with answers.

1. Does Endermologie really work?

Yes, it does, as demonstrated in thousands of case studies from Europe. Similar results are being documented, in photographs and testimonials, in this country by physicians like myself. Ongoing research is being carried out in France, Germany, and the United States to find out exactly how and why it works so effectively.

2. What sensations will I experience during the treatment?

The sensation is similar to deep massage. Most clients find it quite pleasant. The strength of the treatment can be individually adjusted to your personal comfort level.

3. What will I feel afterward?

Most clients report feeling relaxed, with an increased surge of energy.

4. Are there any side effects?

Minor, temporary bruising may occur and should disappear within twenty-four hours.

5. How long does a session last?

Sessions last an average of thirty-five minutes.

6. How many treatments can I have in one week?

The average number is two per week; more than that has not been proven to bring faster results. If you are simultaneously in the process of losing a substantial amount of weight, one treatment a week is recommended.

7. Are my problem areas the only areas worked on?

Problem areas are the focus, but attention is given to other places on the body in order to stimulate general circulation and elimination.

8. How many sessions will it take before I see results?

You will feel better after your first session. Usually people begin to note physical changes within five or six sessions, others by eleven or twelve. The suggested number of treatments is fourteen, but some clients opt for more.

9. What is the cost of treatment?

The price varies nationwide, based on the physician and your individual needs. Typically, a session costs between $85 and $125.

10. Why do I have to drink so much water every day?

The treatments affect the subcutaneous fat layers, helping to release fluids and other waste material that have been trapped by swollen cells. Water is the natural body cleanser that carries away all these impurities.

11. How long do the results last? What about maintenance?

Changes can last for several months up to a few years, depending on the level of physical activity—the more active you are, the better your circulation—and nutrition—low-fat eating is recommended. Once the initial fourteen treatments are finished, you may elect to return on a periodic basis in order to maintain benefits. At the beginning of the maintenance period two sessions per month for two months is recommended. After that, one time a month is suggested. This will, of course, vary from person to person. Some people only require twice-a-year visits to maintain their modifications.

12. How long do I have to wait after liposuction or a tummy tuck to receive a treatment?

Before receiving a treatment, consult with the plastic surgeon who did your tummy tuck or liposuction. Typically, you will have to wait until the compressive garments come off, normally three to four weeks.

13. Does the machine tone skin?

You will likely notice an improvement in skin tone after treatments. The appearance of stretch marks and loose skin may also show improvement.

14. Will I lose weight?

While the machine is not for weight loss, many patients report being able to lose weight more easily while undergoing treatments than they ever could before. Research with obese patients is now taking place in France to study weight loss patterns after a standard course of treatment in the absence of restricted caloric intake or an exercise regimen.

15. What is the difference between Endermologie and liposuction? Can it be used instead of liposuction?

Unlike liposuction, Endermologie is a noninvasive procedure that does not pierce the skin. Instead of liposuction, some people try Endermologie first to see what kind of results they can achieve. Some choose to receive both. Currently Endermologie is being studied and used by some of the world's foremost practitioners of liposuction.

16. Why are photos taken before, during, and after treatment?

Photos are taken to provide an accurate record of improvements. They also help the practitioner to provide better treatments through comparative analysis.

17. I don't want anyone to see my pictures. Is my privacy protected?

No one but your therapist and attendant staff will see your photos. If you wish, you can sign a release that will permit your photos to be used for educational and promotional purposes.

18. Does the treatment work on men?

Definitely. For problem areas such as "love handles" and loose pectoral tissue, the treatments have produced excellent results.

19. Who is not a good candidate for treatment?
See pages 105–106 for the list of conditions that preclude Endermologie.

20. What can I realistically expect?
While it cannot make a body appear twenty years younger, Endermologie can make changes in cellulite and overall skin tone, ranging from subtle to dramatic, depending on age and the state of the skin.

The Cellulite Creams: Do They Work?

American women spend millions of dollars a year on creams, lotions, and other topical applications that yield little, if any, changes, in the appearance of dimply skin. In 1995 alone, sales of anticellulite preparations approached $100 million: Even the promise of a reduction in cellulite is enough to make the most rational woman part with her money.

What's the truth about these "dream" creams? The fact is that, although some manufacturers claim that their products penetrate the skin, breaking down and reducing cellulite, it's just not medically possible. If a chemical were strong enough to keep that promise, it would also damage skin and other body parts with which it were to come into contact.

Some of the more popular cellulite creams contain caffeine as their active ingredient. Others have utilized alpha-hydroxy acids (AHAs), which are derived from milk, sugarcane, and ginger, as well as fruits such as apples, grapefruits, and oranges. Massaged into the offending areas, the AHAs are supposed to act as exfoliants, breaking up and removing the top layer of dead skin, while stimulating the growth of new skin.

Although the skin often looks "rosier," smoother, and softer after the AHAs are applied, this may not be due to improved circulation. The effectiveness of these creams is questionable and, so far, unproven.

The latest cellulite attackers are made with aminophylline, an old standby in asthma treatment. Based on the preliminary findings of two physicians, when aminophylline was applied to the thighs of eleven women taking part in a small research project, it resulted in a barely perceptible amount of shrinkage. In the experiment, each woman received a daily teaspoon of 2 percent aminophylline in a cream base. It was to be used on one thigh for a six-week period. At the end of the test period, the women lost up to a half inch on their treated areas. What caused the very minor losses?

Supposedly, the cream prompted a release of fat cells from the thighs into the bloodstream, which caused the upper leg to shrink in size. However, most researchers now believe that the slight changes were most likely linked to fluid, not fat, loss.

The creams containing aminophylline must be used daily to achieve and maintain any loss. It should be noted that while the researchers used a 2 percent concentration, most commercial creams with this substance contain a 0.5 percent concentration. Instead of promising thigh reduction and cellulite loss, they offer "smoother appearing" thighs. But at upwards of sixty dollars for a few ounces, it seems like a lot of money to pay for so small a return.

Still, even this inconsequential outcome was enough to prompt thousands of women to seek out this newly packaged "cure."

Liposuction: Does It Work on Cellulite?

Liposuction, the removal of fat from the body using a strong suctioning device, is an invasive surgical procedure introduced in this country in 1982. Developed in France, it's now the most common form of cosmetic surgery performed today.

When performed by the hands of a skilled practitioner, liposuction helps to contour and shape the body; it has become the invaluable tool of plastic surgeons who perform both cosmetic and reconstructive surgery.

The procedure is straightforward. For example, removal of fat from the abdomen entails multiple incisions, each no longer than a quarter of an inch. A cannula, a long, thin, blunt-tipped nozzle, is then maneuvered through the layers of fat. By moving the cannula back and forth, the surgeon loosens fat cells, sucking them up through the cannula and into a container. Then the surgeon contours the remaining fat, leaving enough to provide a smooth, even surface.

Having liposuction performed is not to be confused with going to a spa for a massage or a facial. As with any surgical procedure, a thirty- to sixty-minute liposuction session carries some risk. Commonplace as it has become, skin texture can be damaged in some cases, and bleeding and infection is always a possibility. After it's over, most patients are sore for days, and wearing the girdle-like compression shorts for four to six weeks afterward makes many wonder, even momentarily, if it was all worth it.

The procedure is expensive, ranging in price from $1,000 to over $5,000, depending on the surgeon's fees and how many particular sites are treated. Liposuction can be used to remove fat from the legs, buttocks, abdomen, back, arms, neck, and face. But while it offers amazing aesthetic transformations for patients, it is not an instant weight-loss procedure or a cure for obesity. Nor is it a substitute for diet and exercise. Years of experience has shown that liposuction works best for people who are no more than fifteen pounds overweight with taut skin that has the resiliency to snap back into place after fat has been removed. The good news is that, once the fat is removed, it's removed permanently. While you may later gain weight, fat will not accumulate in the treated area.

Unfortunately, liposuction does not remove cellulite. While it can remove deep fat layers, it has less effect on subcutaneous fat layers in the first centimeter under the skin, or on skin tone itself. In many cases where women have liposuction to rid themselves of cellulite, skin texture is actually damaged, resulting in scarring and pitting. Many times second and third surgeries have to be performed to correct the aftereffects of earlier procedures.

Over the years, the array of treatments that have claimed to rid the body of cellulite has ranged from eccentric to potentially dangerous. They include:

- constrictive body wraps to eliminate fluids
- site-specific electric heating pads
- machines that jiggle, pound, and shake the body
- electric stimulation of the muscles
- severely restrictive eating plans

The results are always the same. None of these treatments works to rid the body of cellulite.

Facial Rejuvenation with Laser Skin Resurfacing

No matter how much we exercise or how well we dress, there is one aspect of our body that represents us more than anything else: our face. While genetics, as well as sun exposure, do play a part in how many lines will appear, we can now achieve to a much greater degree an unwrinkled look.

More and more of my patients are opting for rejuvenating facial procedures because they feel that the benefits far outweigh the risks. Today, there are two specific ways to rejuvenate skin without undergoing an invasive surgical procedure: laser skin resurfacing and antiaging cosmeceuticals that feature the latest antioxidant creams and vitamins. I'm in favor of both of them.

The new facial treatments have great advantages: They are noninvasive, cause minimal discomfort, and literally erase years from faces without dramatically altering expression or facial characteristics. The result is a fresher-looking, smoother-skinned face.

This was the case with Helena, a forty-one-year-old

travel agent who was very concerned about her prematurely aging visage.

"I look at my mother, who is in her sixties; she appears at least fifteen years older than she is," Helena told me. "She loves her boat, and the sun is her 'best friend.' I can't say I'm much better. When I was in my twenties, even thirties, I dismissed the thought of using any kind of lotion or sunblock; I liked those tans. But now I look in the mirror and I realize that this weatherbeaten face isn't the real me. I feel great, but my face seems tired and worn. I'm actually concerned that my clients will think I'm too old to sell them the exciting trips that promise to revitalize them and expand their horizons. I want these lines erased."

Helena had originally asked me about having chemical peels; she had read about them in a magazine. I explained that the major problem with having a peel relates to post-peel pigmentation disorders. When it's performed, the doctor puts an acid (such as trichloracetic acid) on the face in order to soften or "peel" away wrinkles, scars, and marks. However, because the acid is applied by hand, the possibility of an uneven, blotchy look is very real.

Instead, I recommended skin resurfacing, using a laser. I referred her to a colleague, a plastic surgeon who uses a special CO_2 (carbon dioxide) laser.

The Carbon Dioxide Laser

The newest technique in cosmetic surgery that is quickly gaining in popularity is carbon-laser resurfacing, a relatively bloodless procedure with a rapid-pulse carbon dioxide laser that can be performed on an outpatient basis. The laser works wonders on a number of skin problems, including wrinkles, acne scars, warts, stretch marks, surgical scars, age spots, and pigmentation changes. The results are similar to those achieved with chemical peels and dermabrasion (a procedure in which a special surgical instrument is used to polish away fine facial wrinkles and scars left by acne)—but with none of the possible complications and side effects of those procedures, which can include scarring as well as discoloration. Using the laser, the risk of scarring and discoloration is less than 1 percent. The procedure can be performed under local anesthetic or with light sedation.

The high power and short pulse of the carbon dioxide laser allow the invisible beam to vaporize the outermost layer of skin on a large area in a matter of minutes. The lasers vaporize water in the epidermal cells—the first layer of skin cells—so that burning of the skin is controlled.

"What the rapid pulse does so well," says plastic surgeon Barry Zide, "is that it allows the surgeon to deliver an exact, calculated amount of energy into the skin in order to remove a thickness of skin without damaging anything else."

Helena's procedure was performed in Dr. Zide's office, which has a small operating theater. Outfitted in a surgical gown and special metal protective glasses, Helena lay comfortably on an operating table. A light sedative was administered to help her relax while Dr. Zide highlighted the areas to be treated with a surgical marking pen.

Holding the laser like a paint brush, Dr. Zide gently stroked away the wrinkles around her eyes and lips. With each tiny zap, the water in her skin cells absorbed the beam, causing the skin to contract and the wrinkles to slowly vaporize. After several minutes, what used to be crow's feet were small, slightly raised red circles. As the procedure continued, Helena's treated areas appeared shiny with the surface skin wiped away. The skin injury she was accepting willingly was the equivalent of a highly controlled second-degree burn.

Postoperative healing can take up to two weeks. In that time, there is plenty of facial oozing and the skin has to be kept moist and clean. Helena was informed of her postlaser regimen and daily makeup technique. As a preventive measure, she also took antiviral and antibiotic medications to reduce the risk of a herpes outbreak or a bacterial infection.

When Helena came to see me six weeks later, she was ecstatic. Her "new" face was still slightly reddened, but she was informed that more than 30 percent of all patients appear sunburned for as long as three to five months after surgery and can wear camouflage makeup until it fades.

"I see a big difference already. That weathered look is gone. I think I look ten years younger—which is how I feel," she said. "I can't get over the difference."

Helena is not the only patient who has had terrific results from laser resurfacing:

• Fran, a fifty-six-year-old nurse, felt like a kid at heart and wanted her face to reflect it. She had her sun-damaged skin corrected, and the wrinkles around her lips and eyes removed. "I bungee-jump, Rollerblade, go snowboarding and skydiving. Why look old and stodgy when I embrace the young and active life?"

• At forty-three, Colin believed that he looked older than his co-workers and had his wrinkles erased. "With all the downsizing at my company I need to look good to compete with the younger crowd, which I hang out with anyway. The more youthful I look, the better reception I get. There is a tremendous stress on appearance in the workplace."

• Ted, at fifty-two the advertising director of his own company, didn't think about his face until person after person remarked that he was looking tired. He certainly wasn't feeling that way—but it made him self-conscious about the wear-and-tear on his face. His wife finally convinced him to do something about it by pointing out that he exercised and ate right in order to look better; why avoid another step that would have dramatic results? He agreed, and had the laser procedure performed on his entire face. Since most men will not use cover-up makeup, a full-face laser job looks more uniform. "I always look relaxed and rested now," he said.

• Gloria, a sixty-one-year-old restaurant owner, doesn't believe in aging gracefully. "It's unfortunate that we're judged on how we look," she says, "but it's a fact of life. I'm so happy with the outcome; it's changed my life."

An Amazing Option

In the past, the elimination of wrinkles required other treatments, depending on what was to be removed. These options included deep chemical peels; collagen injections; dermabrasion, where the outer layers of skin are abraded, or sanded, away; and traditional surgery, where tissue is excised with a scalpel.

Laser skin resurfacing, on the other hand, gives the surgeon very precise control over the exact tissue to be removed, but harm or trauma to underlying or surrounding tissue is minimized. Because of the laser's pinpoint accuracy, it allows the specially trained physician (plastic surgeons and dermatologists typically perform the procedure) to work on areas of the face—close to the eyes, and the upper lip—where other treatments might prove risky. In the right hands, laser skin resurfacing can produce dramatically positive results.

While this procedure is not the only one at a plastic surgeon's disposal, and while it will not be effective for all patients (as I'll explain), it does offer a safe, highly exciting, Vitality Medicine option.

Because laser resurfacing has become a popular procedure with a number of my patients, I have compiled a list of their most asked questions, with answers.

1. Is laser skin resurfacing just the latest fad treatment in plastic surgery?

Absolutely not. Lasers have been used successfully in medicine and this is neither an "experiment" nor a "gimmick." Lasers have been extensively tested and proven in the clinical environment by both plastic surgeons and dermatologists, and those who have used them know what results to expect. Those physicians keep dramatic "before and after" photographs that conclusively show the stunning effects of the procedure.

The carbon dioxide laser system specifically incorporates very advanced, microprocessor-based technology that is specially designed to give the surgeon maximum control. At the same time, thermal damage to underlying and surrounding tissue is minimized.

2. What can laser skin resurfacing do for me?

Understand that the treatment doesn't change the basic

structure and look of your face. What it can do is make your face look younger by eliminating or softening:

- fine wrinkles on the upper lip and forehead
- crow's feet and fine wrinkles around the eyes
- acne scars (variable)
- areas of sun damage and discoloration

3. How do laser treatments compare with collagen injections, chemical peels, and facelifts?

At best, filling wrinkled areas with collagen is only a temporary solution; it must be repeated at regular intervals at a cost of $300 to $500 per injection of a liquid mixture made from the connective tissue of cows or pigs. Collagen-enhanced sites (the upper lip is a prime one) are plumper and cause wrinkles and sagging skin to vanish, but only temporarily. Typically, the effects of an injection last a few months to as long as eighteen months before the body finally breaks it down and reabsorbs the material. Due to its unpredictable nature—the effects of collagen vary due to the individual patient and the part of the face being treated—collagen does not provide so great a cost/benefit ratio as other procedures. However, if you are apprehensive about laser resurfacing and are prepared to repeat the collagen injections on a fairly regular basis, then collagen injections may be the proper choice for you.

Medium-depth chemical peels can remove some finer lines, but they aren't as effective in eliminating more pronounced wrinkles. Deep chemical peels can do a good job of eliminating wrinkles, but they bring a serious problem: There is less control over how much tissue will be removed. Also, deep chemical peels contain phenol, a caustic agent that can cause unwanted, possibly dangerous side effects. And deep peels tend to impart a white, waxy appearance to the skin.

A facelift, or rhytidectomy, is the surgical removal of excess skin, fat, and tissue from the face. The surgery, which is performed by a plastic surgeon, generally takes three to four hours and carries with it all the risks and complications typical with other kinds of surgery, such as bleeding, infection, and problems with anesthesia. Depending on your health and amount of surgery, recovery time can vary from two to four weeks or more. Facial numbness, a common complaint due to the rupturing of nerve endings, is usually temporary, but can last up to a year.

While a facelift certainly can't stop the aging process, it can have a significant effect on the most visible signs of aging—deep creases between the nose and mouth; slack, sagging, and jowly jawline; appearance of folds and fat deposits around the neck. This feat is accomplished when the plastic surgeon removes excess fat and tightens underlying muscles. For some, this enhanced facial appearance can temporarily set your clock back by as much as a decade, making you look younger and fresher. This all depends on your age, how much work is done, the condition of your skin, and the skill of your surgeon.

Of all the procedures I've discussed, a facelift has the potential for the most dramatic change. How long will the "new you" last? Anywhere from five to ten years, say the experts, depending on your genes, as well as cigarette smoke and sun exposure, both of which can speed up skin cell loss. Be sure to discuss fees with your surgeon. Prices vary nationally, depending on the surgeon, but can easily be in excess of $5,000.

4. What are the benefits of laser resurfacing?
There are many, including:

- potentially better results through precise control of the depth, intensity, and placement of the laser beam
- virtually no pain
- no residual "bleaching" of treated skin
- more uniform rapid results

5. Who are the best candidates?
Several factors must be considered when determining if the procedure is appropriate for you. These include your age, medical history, results you desire, and skin type.

While the laser results can be dramatic, this procedure is not for everyone. It is limited, typically, to fair-skinned individuals, the ones who burn before they tan. Those people with mild, moderate, or severe facial wrinkles when their faces are at rest are also good candidates for laser resurfacing.

The procedure is the right option if you:

- fully understand the procedure and are willing to accept the facial oozing and dripping that will follow in the days after the procedure
- are willing to undergo a dramatic change in your daily makeup technique for several months
- will see your doctor three or four times in the first two weeks after the procedure so that your condition can be monitored properly
- are able to take a minimum of two weeks off from work while your face heals

You should be aware that, depending on the specific condition of your skin, more than one laser skin resurfacing may be required to produce optimal effects. Also, in some instances, another plastic surgery procedure, such as a facelift or blepharoplasty (cosmetic eye surgery), may provide better results. Sometimes laser skin resurfacing can be used in conjunction with, or after, a surgical procedure to enhance its effects.

6. What happens before the procedure?

Your surgeon will take a medical history to determine your overall state of health. He or she will want to know if you've been using Retin-A or Accutane (antiacne medication) within the preceding year, or if you've had facial surgery during the previous six months. Prior poor wound healing, keloid scar formation, and extreme sun sensitivity are other factors that will be considered. In cases where hyperpigmentation, an unusual darkening of the skin, is a concern, patients will be given a bleaching agent to use in advance of the procedure. Patients with a history of herpes simplex are given acyclovir five days prior to surgery, and continue taking the medication for a total of fifteen days. If you smoke, your surgeon will advise you to stop for a period of time before and after the surgery; smoking constricts blood vessels, interfering with optimal wound healing.

7. Where is the procedure performed?
In most every case, laser skin resurfacing is an outpatient procedure that requires no hospitalization. If your surgeon does not have his or her own laser, the procedure may be performed at an outpatient surgical center.

8. What goes on during the procedure?
First, you will be given injections of lidocaine, or other local anesthetics, in the facial areas where the laser skin resurfacing will be done. The medication will make your face numb to any stinging, burning, or pain. Your eyes will be protected by special glasses.

Once your face is anesthetized, the work begins. As a safeguard, the laser has a special built-in system that allows the surgeon to confirm that the beam is focused on the area to be treated before performing the procedure.

As skin tissue is removed by the laser, your surgeon will wipe the debris away with gauze soaked in salt water. The entire procedure takes anywhere from fifteen to forty minutes, depending on how much skin surface will be covered. Afterwards, a special cooling dressing will be applied to the treated areas.

9. What can I expect after it's over?
Be prepared: You probably won't want to be seen in public for at least two weeks after the procedure. Having undergone a controlled burn of your face, your skin will be red and yellow, scabbed and swollen, and will ooze for quite some time. It is all part of the normal healing process. After that, the skin is red, and can remain that way for as long as several months.

Oral antibiotics will be prescribed to prevent the chance of infection, which is a risk that accompanies any surgical procedure. You will also be instructed to keep the treated area moist with an antibiotic ointment or petroleum jelly, and to change your dressings often.

Some discomfort is to be expected, and patients may experience a burning sensation after the procedure. To minimize this discomfort, acetaminophen should be taken according to label directions. If stronger pain medication is required, ask your surgeon to prescribe it for you.

Some patients complain of itching; this, too, is normal, but all temptation to scratch the offending sites must be avoided. It can lead to infection and impede the overall results.

After laser skin resurfacing, new collagen forms to replace the damaged layer that has been removed. The new outer layer of skin is composed of healthy new skin, resulting in a smoother, younger-looking appearance. Skin tightening also occurs, the aftereffect of collagen fibers shrinking due to heating the layers of skin below the vaporized areas.

In ten days to two weeks, the area will be resurfaced. After three to five weeks some patients may require depigmenting agents to even the color. Sometimes a cortisone cream is helpful to reduce the redness.

It's very important to remember that you must avoid the sun during the healing process. Even if it's cloudy you will have to put on sunscreen with SPF 15 protection against both UVA and UVB rays. This will help you avoid possible sun damage that can further discolor your skin.

10. How long will the results last?
They seem to last five to six years if you avoid further sun exposure and do not smoke, but additional study is needed. Your surgeon will review your particular skin condition and offer an assessment before you decide to have the procedure.

11. What questions should I ask my prospective surgeon?
Do not decide to undergo laser skin resurfacing until you have asked these questions:

Have you had special laser training?

How long have you been performing laser surgery?

Are you board-certified in this procedure?

May I see before and after photos of previous patients?

What complications have your patients experienced?

How many patients have you treated with this procedure?

Are my skin color and type appropriate?

What side effects should I expect?

May I contact some of your patients who have undergone this procedure?

12. How much does the treatment cost?

It can vary from $1,000 to $4,000 or more, depending on the surgeon's fees, area(s) of your face to be treated, the number of procedures required, the locale of the surgery, and associated charges (such as outpatient facility charges and anesthesia). The perioral (lips and chin) area fees may range from $1,800 to $2,500. The periorbital (around the eyes) fee is in the $1,200 to $1,800 range, with full-face laser costing between $3,500 and $5,500. These costs are regional and vary according to the fee structure of the individual surgeon.

13. Will my health insurance cover laser skin resurfacing?

Unfortunately, no. Since it is considered a cosmetic procedure by insurance companies and managed-care organizations, the patient must pay. The only exception is if the surgery is being used to remove a precancerous skin condition.

14. Are there any new techniques on the horizon?

In the near future, more and more physicians will be switching from the CO_2 laser to the erbium laser, the latest technological advance in resurfacing. Clinical research has shown that the erbium laser is more rapidly absorbed by skin, which means the need for less anesthesia and a marked reduction in reddening of the skin. When using the erbium, recovery times for full-face resurfacing are, in many cases, reduced to a week.

It must be noted that neither the CO_2 nor the erbium laser is meant to remove unwanted facial or body hair. For that, the newly FDA-approved SoftLight laser by Thermolase works quickly, with minimal discomfort, leaving skin soft and smooth.

Like any surgical procedure, laser resurfacing, whether with CO_2 or erbium, demands an informed patient and a skilled surgeon to achieve the best outcome. And while it requires recovery time, the end results can be dramatic. As a Vitality Medicine option, I believe that laser resurfacing offers willing men and women the opportunity to look as young as they feel.

The New World of Cosmeceuticals

When Elisabeth, a forty-year-old ski instructor, came to see me she was practically in tears. "Look at my face. It's leathery and blotchy. And my lips! I've got all these deep lines over my mouth. A few wrinkles are certainly okay with me—but I look years older than my age. Now I realize that everything I heard about unprotected sun exposure is true. Twenty years of sun is on my face and I look haggard. I'm at my physical peak, but my face looks ready to retire. I'm not ready for a facelift and I can't have laser resurfacing because my job keeps me in the sun; I can't take the time to heal properly. What can I do?"

Fortunately, Elisabeth could take advantage of a brand-new world of topical solutions that could improve her skin dramatically. Called cosmeceuticals, these hybrid drug-cosmetic formulations are available without a prescription. They act on the dermis, the dense layer of tissue where skin problems such as wrinkling develop. The dermis, located just below the thinner, outer layer of the skin, is the site of the elastic collagen fibers, those soft and resilient tissues that support the skin and keep it taut. Water, oxygen, and other nutrients travel efficiently through the dermis, nourishing collagen and facilitating excretion of waste products.

Liquid vitamin formulations, and vitamin C in particular, are now available to deliver large amounts of usable nutrients to the skin. When applied on a regular basis, vitamin C helps to erase wrinkles, regenerate the skin, and protect it from further sun-induced damage. Not limiting its use only to people with sun-damaged skin, I also recommend liquid vitamin C to be used preventively on a daily basis to help minimize ongoing damage caused by environmental pollutants.

I told Elisabeth that she was a good candidate for topical vitamin C. In liquid form, Vitamin C has shown excellent results in helping sun-damaged skin by directly repairing collagen that has been destroyed by ultraviolet rays. Its benefits are long-lasting, and if you occasionally forget to put it on, it will still be working. Once applied to the skin, it penetrates the outer layer just enough so that it can't be rubbed, sweated, or washed off. The protective power lasts for at least three days.

I referred Elisabeth to Dr. Jeannette Graf, a former researcher at the National Institutes of Health. A dermatologist in private practice, Dr. Graf has developed her own program utilizing magnesium ascorbyl phosphate, or Mag C, as it's popularly called. Patented by Japanese researchers, Mag C is the most advanced topical vitamin C formulation. It's nonirritating and, when applied twice daily, helps to smooth and firm the skin, leaving it younger looking.

For all patients with excessive wrinkling and extensive patches of sun-damaged skin, carbon laser treatment is surely the better procedure to choose. However, for mild to moderate wrinkling and sun damage, and as a very effective preventive measure for people of all ages, I recommend the cosmeceutical program incorporating Mag C for women and men who want to maintain healthy skin.

Mag C penetrates the epidermis, the outer layer of skin that is only one one-thousandth of an inch thick, delivering more than twenty times the amount of vitamin C found in normal skin. As soon as the concentrated vitamin C is absorbed through the skin, it begins to reduce the sun's damaging effects. Each application protects the skin against future ultraviolet light exposure from both UVA and UVB rays. And it has no side effects.

The improvement in Elisabeth's skin was dramatic and six months later she returned to see me, looking vibrant and happy. "My skin is much smoother, my skin tone is even, and those crow's-feet and lines have really diminished. Even the really deep wrinkles look a lot better. Everyone I know remarks about how great I look. I feel like I've turned back the clock."

Why Our Skin Ages

When we're young, our skin has the ability to resist and repair most of the damage caused by sun exposure and free radicals that attack genetic material in skin cells. However, by the time we're twenty-five, skin begins to lose the battle. Degenerative changes begin slowly but surely, leaving an indelible imprint on the face that, sooner or later, becomes noticeable.

Researchers now know that wrinkles and age spots are not caused by an "aging gene." Today, we realize that the cumulative effects of internal and external factors prevent the skin from duplicating and repairing itself the way it's meant to do. Elements like air pollution, cigarette smoke, and extremes in hot and cold temperatures all contribute to cellular damage. But the major attacks come from ultraviolet A and B rays of sunlight that penetrate the dermis, increasing the free-radical activity in the skin. As the skin is exposed to the sun for longer periods of time, the elastin fibers change and take on the characteristics of a "huge accumulation of tangled, thickened, and strikingly abnormal fibers," as some researchers have described them. Once this occurs, the skin loses its ability to:

- prevent the breakdown of collagen and elastin
- reproduce exact copies of healthy cells
- perform rapid tissue repair

Now, thanks to topical formulations of vitamin C, we have an effective, noninvasive means to combat these ongoing assaults. These preparations have another important function as well: By acting as a mild antiinflammatory agent within the skin cells that received too much sun, they inhibit suppression of the immune system. Researchers believe that this action may also protect against skin cancer, the most common of all cancers.

The Topical Vitamin C Effect

Vitamin C, or ascorbic acid, is vitally important to the skin. It protects against and repairs the negative effects of the sun's rays. But scientists now estimate that at least two-thirds of the vitamin C in the skin is destroyed by ultraviolet light. Since vitamin C is not synthesized in the body and must be provided through diet or supplementation every day, and since we can't utilize more than 1,200 mg daily, cell damage cannot be corrected by supplementation alone.

However, when you apply a pharmacologic level of vitamin C to the skin, in essence feeding it from the outside in liquid form, the digestive tract is sidetracked. Megadoses of the vitamin can be delivered directly to the specific skin site where it is most needed. At these therapeutic levels, researchers now believe that two processes are taking place. Not only is the cosmeceutical interfering with and slowing down free-radical damage to the skin; it is reversing the damage on a cellular level by encouraging new collagen repair and skin regrowth.

The Topical Antioxidant Skin Protection Program

I now recommend to my male and female patients a daily seven-stage program of skin care to help reverse environmental wear-and-tear on the skin and prevent further damage. Do not skip a step. Each one is specifically designed to enhance and improve your skin.

This was the case with Laura and Peter, a couple in their forties who loved outdoor sports and were troubled by their sun-damaged skin. When I explained the regimen to them, Peter was at first resistant. "It sounds like makeup to me," he griped. "I'm not going to use anything I don't feel comfortable about." But Laura was excited about the possibilities of my topical antioxidant skin protection program, and the three of us reached a compromise. Laura would use the program first; if it worked for her, Peter would give it a chance.

A month later Laura called me. "Peter can't get over how much smoother my skin looks and feels. He's convinced—he wants to get started ASAP."

The following scientifically designed program will help your skin repair itself from the assaults of everyday life. Perform it in the morning and evening. To obtain further information about vitamin C and other products call (212) 396-2516.

Step 1: Facial Cleansing. Healthy skin begins with regular cleansing. Gently wash your face using a nonirritating cleanser on your fingers. Avoid using a washcloth or any type of scrub pad or brush; they irritate skin.

Step 2: Mag C Rejuvenation. This specially formulated vitamin C liquid penetrates below the skin's surface, nourishing the skin of your face and neck exactly where it is needed. Place one drop on a fingertip, blending it as far as it will go. Usually about four drops are enough to cover the entire face and neck.

Step 3: Eye Protection—Special Mag C Eye Renewal Cream. The delicate skin around the eyes is the thinnest on the body. Lacking a rich supply of oil glands, this area often appears and feels dry. Place one or two drops of this specially formulated vitamin C cream on a fingertip and apply it around the eye area, avoiding the eyelids.

Step 4: Exfoliation—Beta-Glucaderm Lactate. This is a second lotion to be applied over the liquid Mag C. Composed of alpha-hydroxy acid (AHA), it works to break up the thick outer layer of the skin surface where the buildup of dead, dry cells occurs. The fruit-based acid helps to clean pores, smooth fine lines, and lighten skin discolorations.

The beta-glucans—potent soluble plant fibers derived from oats, barley, mushrooms, and sea life—boost the immune-fighting properties of skin cells. Enabling the cells to defend themselves more effectively against the sun's UVA and UVB rays as well as environmental pollutants, they also stimulate collagen production and help to decrease the depth of lines in the face.

Place one drop on a fingertip, blending the preparation as much as possible; four drops should cover the face and neck. Apply over the vitamin C at night for the first several weeks. Note that you may feel some stinging. This is fine as long as your skin doesn't become irritated. If you have no problem using it every night, begin to put it on in the morning and the evening.

Step 5: Additional Vitamins—Micellular Solution. To further nourish the skin, the Micellular Solution supplies the antioxidants beta-carotene and vitamin E to the surface of the skin. Apply both morning and night following application of vitamin C and beta-glucaderm.

Step 6: Moisturize and Hydrate. Any moisturizer may be applied lightly over the liquid vitamin C treatments. It will work on the skin's surface to trap moisture, keeping it in your skin. Emollients (such as petroleum jelly and mineral oil) work very much like the skin's natural oils. They form a slick barrier on the skin's surface that, to some extent, seals in moisture, thus blocking its evaporation.

The moisturizer that will perform best for you depends on its ingredients and your particular skin type. But the simpler the preparation, the better. The more ingredients present, such as perfumes, colors, thickeners, and emulsifiers, the greater the chance of a sensitivity reaction, especially if you have delicate skin. Be aware that if you are prone to acne, overuse of any moisturizer may prompt a breakout.

Step 7: The Final Touch—Foundation or Sunblock. For maximum protection from the sun, I encourage all of my patients to use foundation with added sunblock after their morning treatment. Foundation cosmetics protect the skin because they contain titanium dioxide, a natural sunblock that wards off wrinkling and blotching. For light coverage, apply with your fingertips.

Sunblock is not just for the summer months; it should be used every day, year-round, as a matter of course. These preparations—creams, lotions, and oils—contain compounds that minimize skin injury by filtering out some or most of the sun's damaging rays. Start using sunblock with an SPF (sun protection factor) of 15. Most contain two or more active ingredients that protect against both types of UV radiation, and most are water-resistant as well.

The New Image Revolution

With these amazing new tools at our disposal, the ability to look and feel as good as you can is a reality. You can rid yourself of cellulite without surgery; erase years off your face with skin laser resurfacing; and repair and protect the skin from sun damage using something as natural as vitamin C. Helping my patients to feel and look as good as they can is one of the most rewarding aspects of Vitality Medicine.

5

Pycnogenol: The Most Powerful Antioxidant Known Today

The use of antioxidants, chemical compounds that neutralize the damaging effects of the cellular by-products called free radicals, has been recognized for years. But when I learned about the long-range benefits of the antioxidant Pycnogenol, I realized that a whole new chapter in Vitality Medicine was about to be written, based in part on this extraordinary pine-bark extract that can prevent or reduce the risk of chronic diseases. An essential component of a complete health strategy and available over the counter, Pycnogenol (pronounced pick-nah-geh-nol) is a patented peak-performance nutrient. It is among the best new weapons I use in my program to maintain overall good health for longer and longer periods of time.

Extending years of optimal health is extremely important because living a competitive, fulfilling existence can have side effects along with great rewards. Sometimes, the very strengths that keep my patients at the top of their game have the potential to backfire, threatening the nonstop energy they depend upon.

Take the case of Peter, a very successful art dealer in his mid-forties, whose normal schedule included flying back and forth to Asia once a month. But suddenly, sitting for hours was beginning to wreak havoc on his back, which had been the source of chronic pain for years. A former college football player, he had developed a mild degenerative disc problem that now seemed to be getting worse. Trying to compensate, Peter had taken up golf and tennis. Typically, he was pushing himself too hard—thirty-six holes on a Sunday morning was not unusual. His wife, familiar with his routine, grew used to helping him out of bed the following Monday.

On a trip to Japan he mentioned his back trouble to a colleague, who told him about a substance called Pycnogenol. The colleague's wife had been using it for a year to treat her arthritis symptoms. Her joint pain had been so reduced that she was now able to return to her daily regimen, which included a two-mile walk, without a hitch.

Peter had been a patient for about three years when he first questioned me about Pycnogenol.

"Frankly," he told me, wincing as he sat down, "I'm ready to try *anything*."

When he mentioned Pycnogenol, I did a thorough search in the medical literature. I discovered that there had been studies on it in France, Germany, and Italy, where laboratory research had been performed to observe how Pycnogenol performed on cells in a test tube, along with animal experiments. So confident were the Europeans of their test results that they were using it in three different ways: as an antioxidant, an antiinflammatory, and an allergy medication.

I told Peter that it was worth trying, especially since the studies supported Pycnogenol's success rate; also, the antiinflammatory medications he had taken in the past had upset his stomach.

Available without a prescription, dosages are determined by body weight, and should be taken twice a day. In Peter's case, that was 300 mg a day, based on 1.5 mg per pound for his two hundred pounds. He took half with breakfast, the other half with lunch.

Less than a week later he called me. "I woke up today without the usual aches and pains. It's such a noticeable difference that I had to tell you right away. I feel like I've been given a reprieve. I'm off to Bangkok tomorrow."

Peter's reaction to Pycnogenol was clear. Working as an antioxidant, Pycnogenol attacked those damaging free-radical molecules that our bodies create every day as a by-product of oxygen use. But it didn't stop there; Pycnogenol also inhibited the release of histamine, enzymes, and prostaglandins that lead to inflammation, thereby helping to relieve Peter's symptoms.

These days Peter is more active than ever. He thoroughly enjoys his sports, and extended flights are no longer a problem. The amazing effects of Pycnogenol have made his active lifestyle pain-free.

Pycnogenol: The New Antioxidant

The protective power of antioxidants has long been recognized by the scientific community. But when I observed the effects of Pycnogenol on my patients, I realized in the most immediate and personal way that an exciting new phase of antioxidant therapy had arrived. Indeed, Pycnogenol has revealed its far-reaching effects in several ways:

• *As a powerful antioxidant:* In 1994 a study at Loma Linda University in California concluded that Pycnogenol can protect endothelial cells (which line the heart as well as blood vessels) from free-radical damage. It went on to propose that Pycnogenol may be utilized to combat corrosive free radicals that are linked to more than fifty diseases, including cancer, which attack the body at the cellular level.

• *As a potent antiinflammatory agent:* Pycnogenol has been shown to reduce the inflammation linked to arthritis, various allergies, and varicose veins by inhibiting the release of enzymes that cause swelling.

• *As a skin protector:* By helping to stabilize collagen, a crucial protein, Pycnogenol promotes improved skin elasticity and smoothness. It also strengthens tiny capillaries, which deliver blood to nourish cells. And, it offers protection against the skin-cancer-causing ultraviolet rays of the sun.

• *As a brain cell shield:* Pycnogenol is one of the few antioxidants that cross the blood-brain barrier. In doing this it protects cells from free-radical damage.

Pycnogenol: What It Is

Neither a vitamin nor an herb, Pycnogenol is a patented formulation of various bioflavonoids extracted from the bark of French pine trees. Flavonoids, derived from plants, are essential nutrients. When the hundreds of known flavonoids are used in the body, they are called bioflavonoids. Each is believed to have a specific biological effect in the body. Vitamin-like compounds naturally found in fruits (especially citrus) and vegetables, seeds, nuts, grains, and soybeans, as well as in cocoa, tea, and wine, flavonoids are our protective allies, battling a host of health ravagers including viruses, cancer, toxic substances, heart disease, and the microorganisms that cause infection. Some are superior to aspirin as platelet inhibitors; others are stronger antioxidants than the famously effective vitamin E.

Pycnogenol, a specific combination of nutrient-packed bioflavonoids, is an incredibly powerful antioxidant. Unlike plant flavonoids, Pycnogenol is water-soluble, which means it is absorbed readily in the body, going to work immediately. It performs a particularly remarkable function by prolonging the quantity of vitamin C in the body. This means that vitamin C, a notable antioxidant in its own right, is able to work longer and harder in the presence of Pycnogenol. It's as if two forces are made stronger by linking up to fight the same battle.

The Pycnogenol/Bioflavonoid Connection

Bioflavonoids act as reliable health protectors. In their natural form they are found in the pulp of citrus fruits. But they are found in other substances as well, such as black tea. For instance, a 1996 Dutch study of 522 men reported that long-term consumption of black tea—the kind that 80 percent of the world and most Americans drink—was linked to a significantly lower risk of suffering a stroke. Researchers point to the flavonoids present in the tea as a possible explanation for the stroke protection.

Flavonoids make blood cell platelets less prone to clotting—in about 80 percent of stroke cases, blood clots block arteries to the brain. The study provided additional information: Those men whose daily intake of tea was high had a 73 percent lower stroke risk than a control group that did not drink the beverage.

Flavonoids also might explain the so-called French paradox. The French, who are consumers of high-fat foods (cheese and foie gras, just to name two), are heavy-duty smokers, and have high concentrations of cholesterol in their blood, nonetheless do not have the problem with heart disease that is rampant in the United States. In France, the typical person still outlives his or her American counterpart by about 2.5 years (76.5 versus 74 years). More impressive, however, is that in spite of their lifestyle behaviors, the French suffer 40 percent fewer heart attacks than their American counterparts. Hence, the paradox.

Several hypotheses have been suggested to explain this, but many researchers now believe there are two reasons:

1. The French drink alcohol with their meals, primarily red wine. High in bioflavonoid content, red wine protects cell membranes against oxidation.
2. In comparison with Americans, the French eat more fresh fruit and vegetables, which contain significant amounts of bioflavonoids.

The problem with adopting the French custom of drinking red wine with lunch and dinner to ward off heart attacks is that it encourages alcohol consumption. And even the most health-conscious eaters don't always derive the full benefits of a balanced diet—which, of course, should include the proper number of servings of fruits and vegetables. Foods lose much of their antioxidant powers once they are frozen, processed, or cooked. Pycnogenol, one of the most potent bioflavonoids ever discovered, can supersede these problems safely and effectively. I have always felt strongly that any preventive nutrient should be as risk-free as possible.

Taking Pycnogenol in conjunction with other specific supplements in my Vitality Medicine program, namely vitamins C and E, will result in good health—and thus a lifestyle boost of very significant proportions.

The Discovery of Pycnogenol

As is true of so much scientific research, the discovery of Pycnogenol was made possible by observation and speculation. In the 1960s, Jacques Masquelier, a French researcher at the University of Quebec, happened upon a particular book. Called *Voyages au Canada,* it related the adventures of the famed explorer and navigator Jacques Cartier in the 1500s. Trapped for the winter on his ship in what is now Montreal, Cartier and his crew suffered, as did many people of the time, from scurvy, caused by a deficiency of vitamin C. Luckily, Cartier's path crossed that of Chief Domagaia, a Native American who had recovered from the ravages of the disease.

Taking branches from a local white pine tree, the chief instructed Cartier to peel off the bark, pound it, and boil it with water and pine needles. The resulting tea was to be drunk several times a day, the leftover boiled leaves rubbed on swollen legs. Within a week, Cartier and his crew were cured.

Masquelier was puzzled and intrigued. He knew that pine needles contained only traces of vitamin C, and the bark none at all. Were the trees actually potent sources of bioflavonoids, the plant substances that have the ability to inhibit the action of certain enzymes that cause inflammation? At the time, he had already begun his own research into bioflavonoids. Determined to find out all he could, he began to test the tree bark in the Quebec area. Soon he isolated the active bioflavonoid components, called proanthocyanidins. His ultimate hypothesis was that the bioflavonoids in the pine bark *enhanced* the vitamin C found in the needles, even in their minute amounts. The combination of the two cured scurvy.

One of the first scientists to isolate, identify, and characterize pine bark proanthocyanidins, Masquelier continued his research after returning to France. There, he discovered that the richest source of proanthocyanidins was the bark of the *Pinus maritima,* the wild pine trees that grow in Les Landes, a region that stretches across the southern coast of France from Bordeaux all the way to the north coast of Spain.

Working with the bark, in 1966 Masquelier extracted a substance he termed "pycnogenol," meaning "substances that deliver condensation products." More than two decades later, Masquelier was granted a patent in the United States for Pycnogenol, a compound he said was beneficial in "preventing the harmful biological effect of free radicals."

The Free-Radical Problem

Since the groundbreaking research over forty years ago by Dr. Denham Harman at the University of Nebraska College of Medicine, scientists have agreed about free radicals. *They strongly believe that free radicals, which are now linked to dozens of deadly diseases, are the greatest contributing factor to aging.*

Highly reactive, oxygen-rich unstable molecules created by normal body processes, free radicals constantly attack organs and tissues. Obliterating cells in their path, mutating DNA, they wreak havoc and weaken our body's defenses, making us susceptible to a number of killers, including cancer and heart disease.

Unfortunately, free radicals are created by abnormal processes outside the body, too. Exposure to hazards such as cigarette smoke, pollution, environmental toxins, exhaust fumes, radiation, and excessive sunlight activate free radicals as well. They trigger the same kind of harm inside our bodies. When we produce free radicals, the process launches a devastating chain reaction in which the killer molecules destroy or maim cells. Attacking membranes and genetic material, corrupting DNA, free radicals violate our mitochondria, the very power centers of our cells.

Think about your exposure to the daily external irritants of everyday life. When the air is particularly polluted—so much so that very young children and the elderly with respiratory problems are advised to stay indoors—how do you feel? Even if you exercise regularly and don't smoke, it's probably a strain to breathe. What if you are seated next to a smoker at a dinner party? It's possible that by the time you get home your throat will be irritated. And let's not forget the effects of a rushed lifestyle. How good do you feel if you don't eat fresh fruits and vegetables every day? Probably sluggish, unfocused, not at your best.

What you are experiencing is free radicals at work. They are scavenging your body, causing a disruption in the very systems that work to keep you healthy.

How Free Radicals Damage

Beginning when we are born and continuing throughout our lives, free-radical damage is created by the complex process by which oxygen is utilized inside cells. Ironically, making free radicals is part of a cell's normal function, which it performs without cease. It is estimated that ten thousand free radicals are produced daily in the body. Unfortunately, all these damaged molecules are missing one or two free electrons, forcing an out-of-control crash into other stable molecules in an attempt to right themselves. Trying to commandeer an electron or two to create an electrical equilibrium, the molecules have now lost any potentially beneficial attributes. Even worse, they have created a dangerous domino effect, destroying other healthy cells as they careen through our systems.

When we're younger, the consequence is relatively minor; the body has an extensive repair mechanism at its disposal to keep cells in working order. However, as we age, the cumulative effects of this unrelenting process begin to take their toll. Cells begin to falter; some die. Brain cells, muscles, and cells in the lens of the eye are particularly vulnerable to attack. Scientists believe that it is the accumulated damage to these cells that leads irrevocably to cataracts, physical aging, and senility. The latest research bears this out:

• Study after study discloses that free radicals increase the risk of all cancers, especially those of the esophagus, stomach, prostate, and colon.

• Free radicals oxidize LDL (low-density lipoprotein) cholesterol on artery walls, causing a buildup of the deadly plaque atherosclerosis, which is the leading cause of heart attacks.

• Free radicals attack the lenses of the eye. Normally clear and colorless, the lens helps to focus light on the retina at the back of the eyeball. Free radicals force the lenses to grow cloudy and opaque, creating cataracts.

• By attacking collagen, the substance that keeps skin moist, smooth, and supple, free radicals cause the breakdown of skin tissues, leading to wrinkles and sagging.

Free to roam throughout our bodies, free radicals have the limitless potential to affect every part negatively. In addition to the conditions it already affects, free-radical damage is now being linked to hypertension, stroke, Alzheimer's disease, leukemia, Parkinson's disease, congestive heart failure, and inflammatory bowel disease.

Pycnogenol vs. Free Radicals

Thankfully, there are steps we can take to fight back. Without these strong countermeasures, free radicals would quickly overrun our bodies, abruptly ending our lives. But while our bodies do have their own built-in defense systems, the ability to combat such a continuous assault is limited.

My weapons of choice are antioxidants, which react with free radicals, neutralizing their detrimental effects. They stabilize the molecule by donating an electron so that the free radical will leave healthy cells alone.

Extensive medical research indicates that increasing intake of certain nutrients, especially vitamins C and E, will help to protect against the ravages of free radicals. Pycnogenol can be a very helpful addition.

A broad-spectrum nutrient with numerous applications, Pycnogenol is unlike any other antioxidant. I choose it frequently to counteract free radicals and enhance the active lives of the men and women who are using my Vitality Medicine program. I've seen Pycnogenol work for my patients time and time again, in a number of different ways:

• *On skin:* When added to the regimen of David, thirty-two, it meant a significant decrease in the severity of his psoriasis, a skin condition marked by scaling and red patches. His itching diminished, and wearing short-sleeved shirts to play racquetball was no longer embarrassing.

• *On blood vessels:* For Kellie, thirty-seven, it meant a reduction of edema, the swelling in her lower legs due to water retention, a condition that began when she became pregnant, and was still noticeable when her daughter was a year old. For the first time in almost two years, her legs were back to their normal shape.

• *On the gastrointestinal system:* For James, forty-three, whose spastic colon flared when his company was downsized and he had to take on more work, it meant fewer distractions due to discomfort.

• *On collagen and elastin:* For Amy, twenty-eight, who loved the sun, it offered protection against damaging rays and, therefore, premature aging.

• *On inflammation:* For Ted, forty-nine, an avid marathon runner, it meant quicker healing from sports-related injuries.

• *On allergies:* For Nick, thirty, it meant relief from the hay fever that plagued him yearly.

Pycnogenol and the Skin

Pycnogenol has had a positive dermatological impact on my patients. When Rosalie came to see me she was certainly healthy on the inside, but the packaging looked wrong to her. At forty-three, a high-level buyer for a fashionable New York store, she was worried and distressed about her face.

"I know these are called laugh lines. Frankly, nothing is *that* funny," she said with a pained smile. Her brow was deeply furrowed, and deep lines radiated down from the corners of her eyes and on both sides of her mouth. Tiny red blotches crisscrossed her cheeks, still faintly visible under the heavy makeup she wore. "What did I do to get this way? I know people older than I am who barely have a line on their faces. Why are my wrinkles so bad?" she asked. "I've got to do something about this—now. My job is all about appearances. I represent my store, and they expect a youthful-looking staff to be their 'front' people. I just can't look worn-out; the younger I look the longer I'll keep my job, and the sooner I'll move up in the organization."

Rosalie confessed that she had two bad habits, both of which had very negative effects on her skin. The first was that she was a two-pack-a-day smoker, the second that she had been a sun seeker all her life.

Exposure to the sun's ultraviolet B (UVB) rays creates wrinkles. The same rays that force your skin to tan also break down collagen and elastin, the structural "cement" that holds skin cells together. Researchers at the University of Michigan have established that just a few minutes of exposure to UVB rays are enough to cause skin cells to make enzymes that break down collagen and elastin, causing skin to wrinkle and sag.

Rosalie knew that smoking was dangerous, but she didn't know just how adversely it affected skin. Smoking thickens and fragments elastin, the long, smooth fibers that give healthy skin its resilience. It also constricts blood vessels that supply oxygen to the skin, drying it out. And it interferes with the body's ability to protect itself against free radicals triggered by tobacco smoke.

Rosalie ultimately decided to undergo laser skin resurfacing to vaporize her wrinkles (see page 114), which I thought was one good solution for her. However, since exposure to UVB rays would continue and she hadn't stopped smoking, I recommended a regular course of Pycnogenol to strengthen and protect her collagen. "It's been suggested that Pycnogenol coats collagen so that it can't be broken down further by free radicals. Think of it as your 'cosmetic pill,'" I told her.

When she came to see me several months later Rosalie was, literally, a new woman. Taut and glowing from the laser work and Pycnogenol use, her skin radiated a newfound youthfulness. "I can't overstate how great I feel—my looks match my life. But I have to tell you—I'm convinced that Pycnogenol has been healing my whole body, from the inside out. And I have a confession to make: I'm still smoking."

Pycnogenol and Smoking

Rosalie hit upon an important point about Pycnogenol, especially as it pertained to her smoking. Ronald R. Watson, Ph.D., a research professor in the Department of Family and Community Medicine at the University of Arizona School of Medicine, recently found that Pycnogenol can provide a significant protective effect for smokers.

In his unpublished research, which was duplicated by scientists in Germany in a much larger published study, Watson tested Pycnogenol on subjects who smoked. Two hours later, he took a blood sample. He knew that smoking caused red cells to clump, blocking arteries and contributing to heart disease. However, the smokers who took Pycnogenol exhibited a fast-acting antiplatelet effect, similar to that of aspirin.

This means that Pycnogenol may offer smokers, and those who come in contact with secondhand smoke, some protection against heart disease. However, be aware that neither Dr. Watson nor I am advocating the continuation of smoking. I have said it before and will keep on restating it: Smoking kills. If you are a smoker, you are paving the way to a possible heart attack as well as a number of loathsome diseases. The toxins in cigarettes are lethal, and there is one simple way to avoid them: Stop smoking.

Pycnogenol and Varicose Veins: An Added Benefit

Varicose veins are a very common condition: It's estimated that 10 percent of American men and 25 percent of American women have them. They can cause discomfort—itching and throbbing are not unusual—but it's how they look that often causes the most pain. While there are medical procedures to deal with them—including "stripping," an invasive technique where the offending veins are, literally, pulled from their sites, and sclerotherapy, another medical option where multiple injections of a solution are used to harden the affected veins and eventually cause them to be absorbed—many of my patients have demanded a better solution.

Pycnogenol has improved the quality of life for a number of my patients and given them the treatment they sought. Joan has been coming to see me for several years. A very attractive woman in her early forties, she has worked hard to achieve success as an executive at a recording company. Healthy and active, she came to my office because she hated the varicose veins that streaked her legs.

"I've looked into the available options," she told me. "But just the thought of veins being yanked from my body makes me sick. And I'll do anything to avoid needles. I feel like I'm marked. My mother has varicose veins and she hates them, too; I can't remember her ever wearing a bathing suit. I've spent years working out in order to keep in shape, but still, these ugly, ropy blue outlines on my legs make me look older than I am and certainly older than I feel. I want them to disappear. Can you help me?"

Along with traditional treatments for varicose veins, which include vein stripping and sclerosing, I suggested she supplement with Pycnogenol. Joan began a regimen appropriate to her weight, and five months later the effects were noticeable: Her skin was smoother and the veins were much less visible. Now she proudly wears shorts and bathing suits to show off her toned legs.

"I can't get over the difference," she exclaimed. "Short skirts are the 'uniform' at work, and I'm so comfortable in them now. I don't need to wear pants or dark, opaque tights to cover up my legs. And frankly—my legs are better than those of a lot of twenty-five-year-olds in my office!"

Another of my patients was able to showcase the effects of Pycnogenol. Richard, a highly successful magazine writer in his fifties, had had varicose veins for years. Dressed for work, he wasn't bothered that much about the appearance of his legs. But he did avoid shorts in the summer. His biggest problem, however, was at the end of a long day in front of the computer. That was when his legs ached and itched unbearably.

"I thought that losing weight would have helped," he told me. Formerly weighing in at 280 pounds, far too heavy for his five-foot nine-inch frame, he had slimmed down considerably. But years of sitting and carrying extra pounds had caused his veins to lose their natural elasticity, leading ultimately to the visible blue bulges just beneath his skin. Ironically, losing weight had brought the varicose veins closer to the skin's surface.

I explained that the way veins are constructed and function had a lot to do with his problem. The pumping action of leg muscles pushes blood through a collection of veins on the surface of the muscles, which in turn are connected to deeply imbedded blood vessels. When a muscle relaxes, these veins expand, drawing blood from the superficial vessels. All the interior veins have one-way valves that prevent blood from flowing back into the surface veins. Fragile, thin-walled, and hollow, with little elasticity and muscle, veins have tiny folds of tissue that serve as valves in their inner walls. These valves open when blood flowing upward pushes through and close if blood from above falls back, ensuring a one-way passage.

But when we don't pump our leg muscles, the valves can't fight the force of gravity, and the volume of blood in the surface veins increases, along with pressure, resulting in twisted and dilated vessels. Eventually varicose veins begin to form.

I told Richard that there were several options for dealing with them. One was the vein-stripping procedure that he was familiar with; his wife had undergone the surgery several years earlier after the birth of their third child. "I'm looking for a solution without surgery," he told me.

Pycnogenol was the answer. A 1989 Italian study of forty people with varicose veins showed that taking 100 mg three times daily was enough for marked improvement. Also, I advised Richard that moving around more was very important. Sitting for hours forced blood to pool in his lower legs; walking and leg exercises got his calf muscles pumping, and blood flowing in his veins.

Three weeks after instituting a program that included Pycnogenol, he called me. "The itching is gone," he reported. "And that end-of-the-day throbbing has really diminished."

Two months later, a follow-up visit showed that the gnarled, ropy outline of his veins had smoothed considerably. Richard is taking his Pycnogenol, feels great, and is more productive than ever.

Pycnogenol and Cardiovascular Disease

Most of my patients are well informed about health risks, and even though they work to maintain their vitality they often express concern about specific debilitating diseases. Together with cancer, heart disease is the condition I am most often asked about.

I can readily understand why. Affecting more than 70 million Americans, cardiovascular disease—which includes heart disease, stroke, angina, hypertension, and arrhythmias—is the number-one killer in this country. It is caused primarily by atherosclerosis, a condition in which arteries are clogged with deposits of plaque, which consists of fats such as cholesterol, fibrous tissue, and other substances found in the blood.

The first step in this destructive process is the depositing of cholesterol on arterial walls. Carried through the bloodstream on a group of proteins called lipoproteins, most cholesterol is transported on low-density lipoprotein, or LDL (this is the "bad" cholesterol). On the other hand, HDL, or high-density lipoprotein, the "good" cholesterol, carries less cholesterol than LDL. Once LDL cholesterol is deposited on arterial walls, the damage begins.

The process takes years, but young people can be carrying the potential for deadly heart disease long before symptoms are noticed. Autopsies of almost 80 percent of the healthy, young American soldiers killed during the Korean War revealed major signs of atherosclerosis, mostly caused by a fat-rich diet. Korean soldiers, however, whose diet consisted mainly of rice and vegetables, showed no signs whatsoever of the condition when their autopsies were performed. This study reemphasizes the essential relationship between diet and heart disease.

Over years, plaque builds up, hardening or calcifying. As a result, arteries lose their elasticity, and a section of plaque may break off, creating a clot that can lead to a heart attack. However, while atherosclerosis is not reversible, it can be stopped at any stage, thereby putting the brakes on further artery damage.

Pycnogenol does this:

• It helps the body neutralize free radicals. Free radicals oxidize LDL cholesterol and increase its destructive effects on arteries.

• It keeps blood platelets from becoming sticky as they pass through narrowed arteries, therefore preventing them from clotting at plaque sites.

• It protects the endothelium (the cells of the heart lining), thereby reducing the formation of blood clots that can lead to a heart attack.

• It decreases blood pressure by inhibiting the formation of angiotensin, a substance in the blood that constricts vessels. Animal studies with Pycnogenol conducted in Hungary revealed a pronounced decrease in both systolic and diastolic blood pressures. And new research is beginning to show that Pycnogenol may assist in lowering blood pressure (or hypertension) without the adverse side effects common to many antihypertensive drugs.

Pycnogenol and the Immune System

A highly effective immune system is our best defense against injury and disease. Constantly on alert, this complex system selectively seeks out, recognizes potentially harmful elements (and files them away for future reference), and defends our bodies by:

- fighting off invading germs and viruses, and therefore infections
- counteracting carcinogens, and therefore cancer
- inhibiting allergens, and therefore allergies

When it is working at optimum levels, the immune system—comprising lymphocytes (white blood cells), bone marrow, lymph nodes, spleen, thymus gland, tonsils, and appendix—keeps our bodies in solid working order.

Nevertheless, even the most efficient system can always use extra help. Pycnogenol has been shown to boost the activity of natural killer, or NK, cells. Research carried out by Dr. Ronald R. Watson at the University of Arizona in 1995 clearly indicates that Pycnogenol significantly increases the activity of these powerful cells. Packed with granules filled with lethal chemicals, NK cells attack the body's enemies, killing on contact. In Watson's study, conducted on female mice, one group was inoculated with a retrovirus infection similar to the human AIDS virus. Another group was given ethanol to drink along with their food. Control groups were then set up using normal, uninfected mice. Not surprisingly, an immune deficiency caused by the virus and the alcohol was immediately observed. However, when Pycnogenol was introduced, it dramatically increased the immune response of the NK cells, helping to normalize the activity that had been lost due to the infection and the alcohol.

The Pycnogenol Program

Pycnogenol should be taken daily as part of an overall preventive antioxidant program. To receive maximum benefits, I prescribe a unique two-phase schedule that ensures optimal benefits. The first part is called the saturation phase, the second the maintenance phase.

To begin, the saturation dose schedule is followed for ten days. I recommend that Pycnogenol be taken twice daily with meals so that it can be absorbed with food. For this phase, the most effective dosage is 1.5 mg per pound of body weight daily. For example, a 140-pound person would use 210 mg every day during this period.

At this dosage, within two days you may begin to experience some relief from chronic problems you may have, such as arthritis. If, however, the condition is acute, I recommend that the saturation dosage be continued for as long as one to three months. (For instance, I have had some patients with arthritis maintain the higher dosage for six months. But, once satisfactory improvement was experienced, the dosage was gradually reduced to the maintenance level.)

The maintenance phase is determined after consultation between the patient and his or her doctor. During the maintenance phase, the dosage is halved. This is the amount of Pycnogenol necessary to ensure continued maximum effectiveness. Simply cut the saturation dose in half, and continue to take the new amount twice a day with meals.

The Safety Factor

Pycnogenol studies carried out at the Pasteur Institute in Lyon, France, have shown it to be nontoxic to humans. In one study, daily doses of up to 35,000 mg were given for six months, with no adverse effects. Pycnogenol should be viewed as a completely safe nutrient.

Pycnogenol Guidelines

• Inform your doctor that you are thinking of taking Pycnogenol. Although there are no known drug interactions, for your own protection it's always prudent to keep your physician up to date about all vitamins and supplements you are taking.

• Purchase Pycnogenol®, a patented nutrient and a registered trademark of Horphag Research Limited. Be aware: There are imitators who use the name illegally. However, buying Pycnogenol with this trademark assures that the nutrient is manufactured exclusively from the bark of maritime pine trees from coastal France. It guarantees as well that the Pycnogenol contains up to 95 percent pure proanthocyanidins (nontoxic, water-soluble antioxidants), and contains no solvent residues, natural or synthetic additives, or other dilutants.

• Check the expiration date. Because Pycnogenol is one of the best-selling supplements in this country, freshness is usually assured. However, to make sure that you have the best supply possible, check that the expiration date is at least a year away from the date of purchase.

• Use Pycnogenol at mealtimes. It is best absorbed when taken with food.

• Take Pycnogenol every day according to the dosage schedule to ensure its full benefits. Research has shown that taking it at therapeutic levels is necessary to attain the best results.

6

Twenty-first-century Heart Protection Is Here Now

My patients, knowledgeable about the major risk factors for heart disease, are aware of the dangers of high cholesterol levels, carrying too much weight, smoking, high blood pressure, and not exercising. Most live a healthy lifestyle, but they are concerned about what they read and hear about heart disease. Many of their hard-driven colleagues have been felled by heart attacks at a young age. They continually ask about new developments in cardiac protection, and, as a part of my Vitality Medicine program, I can provide them with the latest technological innovations. Now, evaluation is more accurate, heart-protective measures can be instituted, and patients can be reassured— sooner than ever before.

The cardiac prevention program that I have put together will give you many new insights on individualized heart care, as well as specific tests and technologies for both men and women to help protect their hearts against disease.

Detection and Prevention: The Heart's Best Defenses

When it comes to cardiac care I have one specific goal: detection of a condition in its earliest stages before it can become heart damaging and life-threatening. Doctors now have new diagnostic tools that give us an up-close-and-personal look into our patients' hearts, permitting us to see potential—or established—conditions. This means that treatments can begin before an event takes place. And it means that a high quality of life, and the peak performance that accompanies it, can be maintained and extended.

Along with traditional modalities, Vitality Medicine employs several different implements to do this. They are the Ultrafast CT Scan, the Heart Rate Monitor, the Cardiophone, Female-Specific Heart Screening, my stress management technique called S.A.V.E., and cardioprotective nutrients and supplements. All can be used to combat a deadly foe before it takes over our hearts, our vitality, and our lives.

The Statistics Today

Heart disease is the biggest health enemy we have: Coronary artery disease (CAD) due to atherosclerosis is the number-one cause of death in this country, killing 650,000 men and women annually. One in six of all men will experience a heart attack before the age of sixty-five. Although traditionally viewed as the "widow maker," heart disease is now the number-one killer of women, and preventive steps must be taken much earlier to ensure maximum heart health.

Atherosclerosis, often referred to as "hardening of the arteries," is a medical term for a dangerous condition in which arteries are first narrowed and then clogged with plaque, leading to a heart attack. Atherosclerosis—from the Greek "atheroma" for bulge and "sclerotic" for hardening—builds up over years, aided by smoking, high blood cholesterol, or hypertension. Even more frightening, however, is the fact that 300,000 deaths occur suddenly, without the typical warning signs—uncomfortable pressure, tightness, or a burning pain in the chest, or shortness of breath.

A particularly sobering fact is that in eight out of ten cases of seemingly healthy people who die unexpectedly, the cause is a severe plaque blockage of one or more of the major coronary arteries. In fact, it is now recognized that the presence of coronary artery plaque is a more accurate predictor of heart attack than all other risk factors combined, including cholesterol levels and chest pain.

Even more troubling is the fact that fatal heart attacks can happen in people who don't develop a large accumulation of plaque. Instead, they have a thin layer of plaque that coats their arteries. Serious problems arise when this plaque "cracks." A hemorrhage occurs at the site, blocking the artery and quickly resulting in a heart attack.

I want to ensure that my patients have the best protection possible when it comes to their hearts, and that they have no surprises or regrets. Today, doctors have a new coronary artery screening test that is able to detect the indication of heart disease. This means that positive early actions can be taken—whether they are lifestyle changes or medication use—to prevent an attack from occurring by reversing or controlling the course of heart disease.

The diagnostic test that quickly and painlessly tells doctors and patients if trouble is brewing is a critical component of my Vitality Medicine program. It is called the Ultrafast CT Scan.

The Ultrafast CT Scan

A noninvasive test that can predict the likelihood of suffering a heart attack long before the event can happen, the Ultrafast CT Scan detects and locates calcium deposits—not plaque—in coronary arteries. The calcium is found within the plaque, but doesn't cause it. Rather, it is a red flag: Researchers have discovered that the mere presence of calcium in the heart is one of the earliest indicators of progressive coronary artery disease. Having this information is vital because just looking at cholesterol levels can't give you or your doctor the most accurate data about your heart. For instance, you can have low cholesterol levels and still have calcium, the plaque marker, in your heart's blood vessels. And you can have high cholesterol readings while the test shows that you have no coronary plaque at all.

The point is this: *No cholesterol number, no matter how low, is a guarantee that you are immune to heart disease.* With the definitive Ultrafast CT Scan, doctors can take a giant step in coronary prevention.

Armed with lifesaving information, a physician can begin to work aggressively with patients, male and female, to prevent heart damage. While the calcium within the arteries is only a signal of the presence of heart disease, and not a risk factor in and of itself, other cardiac risk factors can certainly be reduced. Lifestyle changes might include an adhered-to low-fat diet bolstered with a regular exercise program, further enhanced with a regimen of heart-protective supplements (see page 192). If indicated, the new cholesterol-lowering statin medications may be prescribed. Then, three to five years after these measures are enacted (and perhaps sooner, if studies currently being undertaken prove this to be true), the doctor will advise a follow-up CT Scan to see how much progress has been made in halting the deadly progression of atherosclerosis.

The Ultrafast CT Scan: How It Works

Developed in the 1980s, the scan is a very rapid computed tomography X-ray twenty times faster than the normal CT. It is this very speed that makes it possible to take computer images of the pumping heart, exposing any calcium buildup in the coronary arteries. The accumulation of calcium in the coronary arteries is a marker for—not a cause of—atherosclerosis and is not linked to the intake of milk, milk products, or calcium supplements.

The angiogram is the only other comparable test that offers a view of the heart that can identify the presence of atherosclerosis with a higher degree of accuracy. Unfortunately, the angiogram, an invasive view into the arteries, requires an anesthetic and a minimum hospital stay of at least half a day. While the incidence is very low in experienced hands, the procedure has potential side effects, including blood clots, stroke, blood vessel injury, and heart attack. In addition, this method of detection often carries with it a considerable four-figure price tag.

"The Ultrafast CT test is the state-of-the-art screening device at this time," states Dr. Alan Guerci, who heads the heart-testing program at St. Francis Hospital in Roslyn, New York. This facility is the only one in the New York metropolitan area—and only one of the thirty hospitals in the United States—to have the machine at this time.

St. Francis installed their $2 million scanner in 1993, and since then Dr. Guerci has instituted an aggressive testing program that attracts patients from around the world. He has also authored several peer-reviewed studies on the Ultrafast CT technology and its specific applications in heart disease detection. In one study of 1,185 patients with scan-detected calcifications but no other symptoms of heart disease, Dr. Guerci found a direct link between the degree of calcification and the likelihood of impending heart attack or stroke.

Coronary artery disease is the most common and also the most expensive medical condition in this country, costing an estimated $60 billion annually. "But by identifying and assessing all known risk factors at a much earlier stage with the CT Scan," said Dr. Guerci, "intervening when necessary, you can then help reduce this human and economic toll."

How the Test Works: Four Patients' Histories

Jake's Story

When I recommend that a patient have an Ultrafast CT Scan performed, the reaction is inevitably, "What's that?" Because the test is so new and not yet generally prescribed, most patients need to learn more about it before deciding to go forward. However, once they see the results, they are impressed by its accuracy and simplicity and are uniformly supportive of the test.

This was the case with Jake, a baseball coach who was, at fifty-one, concerned about his family's cardiac history as well as his own health. He had reason to come to me. His father had first suffered a heart attack when he was forty-seven years old, and succumbed to a massive cardiac arrest nine years later. On his mother's side, Jake could recount a number of relatives who suffered with heart disease. And even though he was an avid bicyclist and carried his 180 pounds on his six-foot-one frame quite well, his blood tests were troubling. His cholesterol was 260 mg/dl—way above the desirable 200 mg/dl or below—and his HDL cholesterol was 30 mg/dl, way short of the protective level of 60 mg/dl, which put him at an increased risk for coronary artery disease. His triglycerides, the main form of fat found in the human body, were 290, well above the maximally desirable level of 200.

These cardiac risk factors, coupled with his inability to lower his cholesterol, impelled me to recommend a course of the cholesterol-lowering statin medications. These drugs, including Mevacor, Pravachol, Zocor, and Lescol, are basically the same, well-tolerated, and both cost- and medically effective. They can dramatically reduce cholesterol by blocking production of a key enzyme needed to manufacture lipoproteins. With the drop in lipoproteins, especially the dangerous low-density (LDL) type, comes a reduction in fat-filled plaque.

Jake, however, was reluctant to use the drugs. "You're telling me that not only are the drugs expensive—a thousand dollars a year is a lot of money—but you're also saying that I'll have to take them for the rest of my life. Yes, I'm concerned about my health—but I'm fifty-one years old and I want more proof," he told me. It was at this juncture that I informed him about the benefits of the Ultrafast CT Scan, suggesting that we hold off the final decision on the statin regimen until we had his test results back.

The Test: Jake went to St. Francis Hospital, where he was tested without even having to change out of his suit. He was surprised at this, but clothing doesn't interfere with this new technology. He was asked to lie down on a table; then he was slowly rolled under a doughnut-shaped ring that took multiple X-rays of his heart—a relatively small six-inch area—at the rate of one every one-tenth of a second. At that speed, the scan "froze" his beating heart, allowing for the detection of calcium in the coronary arteries. A mere five minutes later, the test was over.

Jake watched as Dr. Guerci called up the pictures on his large monitor and began to compute the calcium score. The final tabulation was obtained by comparing the amount of calcium detected in Jake's heart to norms that have been established for men his age from studies of over three thousand heart patients.

The following day in my office, standing halfway across the room, I could see the white spots standing out prominently against the gray tones of Jake's overall heart picture. These calcium markers, I told Jake, were indicators of coronary artery disease. It turned out that his readings were above average for a man his age. The test demonstrated that not only was Jake at risk for atherosclerosis, but actually showed evidence of significant atherosclerosis. Fortunately, the deposits were highly treatable at this stage with cholesterol-lowering medication.

"Seeing is believing," said Jake, staring at the screen. "I don't want to have any surprises or regrets. I'll take my medicine—and I'll really watch my diet from now on. And I'll initiate my fitness program in earnest."

Jake kept his word. He began taking his daily statin medication to lower his cholesterol and eliminated the fat-laden foods in his diet. Within six months his cholesterol reading dropped to 172, his HDL was 48, his triglycerides 180. He lost seven pounds, but, more significantly, his percentage of body fat fell from a decent 24 percent to a much healthier 18 percent.

Jake now admits that the calcium score he received from his Ultrafast CT test was the turning point that made it possible to enact the beneficial risk-reducing behaviors that he did. This phenomenon—responding positively only in the presence of hard data—is one I have noticed with many of my patients. The need for physical evidence in order to motivate lifestyle change is one that was recently documented in an *American Journal of Cardiology* study of over seven hundred men and women.

Dorothy's Story

Dorothy, a fifty-five-year-old librarian, loved spending time with her grandchildren. But she was exceptionally worried that a sudden heart attack would kill her, since she was aware that the risk of coronary artery disease increased significantly in the postmenopausal period. She had no family history of heart disease; rather, her concern was based on a high cholesterol count of 280. An unusual aspect of her case was that because she was underweight, her food consumption did not seem related to her elevated cholesterol level. Eliminating any more fat from her diet was tricky; I had to be careful not to strip her nutritionally because she had a difficult time maintaining her weight as it was.

Dorothy also had a high HDL level and a low triglyceride level, both good heart signs, and she was following through with hormone replacement therapy. But her fear of heart disease was limiting her zest for life.

I recommended the Ultrafast CT Scan to determine whether her elevated cholesterol levels were associated with coronary artery disease, or were merely a genetic anomaly.

Dorothy agreed to take the test and was both delighted and relieved with the results: No calcium showed up on her test, a significant finding because, in her age group, some plaque buildup was expected—regardless of cholesterol levels. Happily, I told her to just come in for her periodic checkup so that I could monitor her vitality markers.

Harriet's Story

At fifty-eight, Harriet, a junior college teacher, had only one health problem. She complained of a fatigue that developed soon after she awoke and became more pronounced as the day went on. Instinctively she felt that something was not right.

"I have no energy," she told me. "The simplest household chores knock me out. This just isn't like me—and I want to know what's wrong so that we can fix it."

I was concerned that Harriet's one symptom, fatigue, was a coronary artery disease indicator. I have seen a number of patients with critical coronary disease who told me that, for a period of several months before their problem was diagnosed, they had no energy and felt washed out. They'd wake up in the morning and feel fine, but as the day went on, they'd try to do something but feel exhausted for hours afterwards.

Harriet's thorough workup included an Ultrafast CT Scan. Her test results revealed a serious heart condition, indicating that an immediate angiogram was necessary. It turned out that she had an almost complete blockage of the left anterior descending coronary artery.

I saw Harriet a month later after she underwent a successful balloon angioplasty procedure to correct the damage. She was then placed on my cardioprotective program, which I suggested she follow for the rest of her life.

Saul's Story

Saul, a hard-driving labor negotiator, had his first crippling heart attack when he was fifty. He was recently divorced and still hadn't gotten over his anger. There were other problems, too. Saul had stopped taking his cholesterol-lowering medicine and daily aspirin and was flirting with disaster.

"For the last three months I've been aware of changes when I exercise," he told me. "I feel some vague chest pains, and I get so tired that I've had to cut my golf game back from eighteen holes to nine; even a set of doubles tennis wipes me out. And I don't even want to talk about what the job stress is doing to me. But to tell you the truth, I'm here because I twisted my knee and I'm having trouble walking."

Saul's knee problem was a simple ligament strain, but his heart condition was much more serious. He needed an immediate workup for his cardiac condition. Concerned that in Saul's case, his predisposition to high cholesterol might indicate plaque buildup, I wanted him to start a course of heart-protective vitamins and nutrients as well as to start taking his statin drugs and aspirin once again. Also, I suggested that he begin my stress management technique (see page 190) to help defuse his daily work-related tensions.

Saul understood the value of dealing with his stress, but he balked at the idea of becoming, as he called it, "drug dependent." "I can get my cholesterol down without drugs—I know I can. Besides, I think I get enough vitamins in the food I eat."

Since Saul had trouble walking and couldn't take a traditional treadmill stress test, I scheduled him for his first Ultrafast CT Scan. It showed that he had a significantly high coronary calcium score that foreshadowed another, perhaps more devastating, heart attack. I explained that the test indicated the need to go beyond statin drugs and have an angiogram performed. After I consulted with Saul's cardiologist, based on his symptoms and Ultrafast CT Scan results, our patient was admitted to the NYU Medical Center for the procedure. This additional test revealed severe coronary disease requiring a bypass, which was performed successfully.

"I guess I can't always negotiate or will myself into a better position," he later told me. "I was sicker than I let on; I was more than a little out of breath. But now I've been given a second chance—I have to take advantage of it."

Now on a cardioprotective program that includes diet, exercise, supplements, and my S.A.V.E. stress-management program (see Chapter 6), as well as regular monitoring by his cardiologist, Saul also makes use of a new device that lets him self-monitor the stress on his heart. We'll talk about this innovative and lifesaving device later on in this chapter.

How Other Tests Compare

When Larry, a forty-nine-year-old carpet dealer, came to see me, he was scared. His longtime business partner—only a few years older than Larry—had just suffered a fatal heart attack.

"Could you prescribe a treadmill stress test for me?" he asked. "I need the peace of mind to know that not exercising—which I haven't done since I was discharged from the army twenty years ago—won't kill me."

I informed him that the lack of exercise was a risk factor for heart disease but that I wasn't in favor of routine **exercise stress testing.** Although it is one of several techniques used to detect cardiac problems, and is often used as a screening device for people about to begin an exercise program, the test is considered too unreliable to provide solid information about people with no cardiac symptoms, such as chest pains or shortness of breath. It may also suggest heart problems where they do not exist, especially in women under the age of fifty. Additionally, if someone is taking medication that affects blood pressure or heart rate, those drugs can alter the outcome of the stress test. (The Ultrafast CT Scan is not affected by drugs.)

Also, stress testing cannot reliably detect what cardiologists refer to as nonobstructive coronary disease. These are the significant blockages, the narrowing of the arteries that have not yet begun to cause trouble. Most stress tests can detect a narrowing of a coronary artery when it is greater than 50 percent. While this is certainly good, it's just not good enough. Some researchers have shown that in many cases of a coronary artery narrowing leading to heart attack and sudden death, the severity of the narrowing is in the 30-to-50-percent range.

However, here's the exciting news: *While a stress test is unable to pick up virtually any of these less-obstructed coronary arteries, the Ultrafast CT Scan will detect most of these earlier plaque deposits.*

Exercise testing on a treadmill or bicycle is a standard medical procedure. It measures how your heart and blood vessels respond to gradually increasing exercise intensity, something that a "resting" electrocardiogram (EKG) cannot do. Many people over forty often worry about the risk of a heart attack during or after exercise; to them, it seems logical to undergo an exercise stress test. But medical decision making is never that easy.

While the stress test itself poses few health risks, is noninvasive, readily available, and costs between $250 to $300, the results are frequently inconclusive. In far too many instances, exercise testing of people with no signs of heart disease registers a false-positive reading—erroneously indicating heart disease. This can happen to as many as 10 percent of people who are tested, resulting in needless anxiety as well as additional heart testing.

Exercise testing can only detect advanced coronary artery disease. In fact, because of its inability to detect early heart conditions, the American Heart Association does not recommend this test for routine screening of persons who have no coronary symptoms.

If you don't have any injury or chronic illness that could keep you from exercising, a more reliable test called a **thallium perfusion scan** is typically ordered to help determine if any areas of the heart are not receiving adequate blood flow. In this procedure, following an exercise stress test, the radionuclide thallium-201 is administered intravenously while the patient runs on a treadmill. A special camera then shows how the thallium is circulated in the heart. While this test is more precise than an exercise stress test (it is rarely false-positive), it cannot detect early coronary artery disease, takes five hours, and costs three times as much as the Ultrafast CT—upwards of $1,200.

Should a significant abnormality show up in this test, a **coronary angiogram** is usually recommended. This entails having a thirty-two-inch-long catheter inserted into the artery in the groin and moved up until it reaches the heart. Dye is then injected into the coronary arteries and X-rays are taken to look for any blockages that may be present. While cardiac catheterization is the most reliable diagnostic heart test, it carries a one-in-one-thousand risk of arterial damage, heart attack, stroke, and even death. It is also the most expensive, costing between $3,000 and $4,000.

A less commonly used test is called the **stress echocardiogram**. When it is performed, ultrasound pictures of the heart are taken before exercising. First the patient walks on a treadmill at progressively increasing speeds while blood pressure and heart rates are monitored. Then the person quickly lies down on the ultrasound table, so that pictures of the still rapidly beating heart can be obtained a minute after exercise ceases. The plus of this test is that it has more precision than the stress test in finding specific areas of the heart that have impaired blood flow. The minus is that it costs twice as much as an Ultrafast CT Scan (approximately $750) and cannot detect early coronary disease.

To give Larry the peace of mind he needed, I recommended that he have an Ultrafast CT Scan. After he passed his test with flying colors—his readings were a perfect zero for calcification—I set up an appointment for him with a fitness trainer. A comprehensive fitness program was designed for him, combining aerobic exercise and resistance training. In the following year, the regimen would gradually and safely bring Larry to the highest levels of fitness. He now exercises four times a week for a minimum of thirty minutes at each session.

Altering Your Cardiac Destiny

As the ultimate noninvasive diagnostic cardiac tool, the Ultrafast CT Scan has the potential to become the "heart's mammogram" by helping to diagnose early heart disease and preventing it from becoming a deadly killer. Here is a list of the most frequently asked questions about the Ultrafast CT Scan, with answers.

1. How does the Ultrafast CT Scanner work?
It uses electron beam technology, which has been in use in radiology for more than ten years and is proven to be safe (radiation exposure is equivalent to two chest X-rays or one abdominal X-ray).

2. How accurate is the Ultrafast CT Scanner?
It is able to detect early coronary disease 85 percent of the time and advanced coronary artery disease 95 percent of the time. It is particularly effective for men over the age of forty, and women over the age of fifty. In most patients over the age of fifty, the rate soars to nearly 100 percent accu-

racy (calcium tends to be found in larger amounts in older plaque).

3. Who should have an Ultrafast CT Scan?

The earlier you diagnose a cardiac condition and initiate a cardioprotective program, the better off you are. Candidates include men between the ages of forty and seventy and women between the ages of fifty and seventy with one or more of the following risk factors for heart disease:

- cigarette smoking
- diabetes
- elevated cholesterol level
- family history of heart disease (sudden death, heart attack, or need for angioplasty or bypass surgery) in a first-degree male relative (parents or siblings) fifty-five years old or less, or a first-degree female relative sixty-five years old or less.
- high blood pressure
- obesity
- sedentary lifestyle

If you have multiple risk factors, or one particularly severe risk factor, you need to talk to your physician about earlier intervention. For example, if you are a thirty-five-year-old male and your father died at the age of forty-one of a heart attack, I would recommend that you have an Ultrafast CT Scan.

4. What if my test shows calcification?

It indicates the presence of some coronary disease, with the amount directly related to the progress of the condition. A high score, where considerable calcium is detected, suggests a moderate-to-high risk of a heart attack occurring within the next two to five years.

5. What if my test shows no calcification?

This means that you probably don't have any coronary disease, and that your likelihood of having a heart attack is extremely low. You may need to work on any modifiable risk factor. For now, relax, and plan on scheduling another test within the next three to six years.

6. Is it reasonable that I have the test performed if I don't have any risk factors for heart disease?

Absolutely. A number of my patients are having the scan performed strictly for preventive reasons as part of my early detection program. Even though there are quite a few who end up with zero or very low calcium scores, the scans have also picked up coronary artery disease in quite a few asymptomatic patients. According to Dr. Guerci, more than 10 percent of patients (men over forty and women over fifty) with no known risk factors have gone to St. Francis Hospital for testing on their own, and have shown alarmingly high coronary calcium scores.

I explain to my patients that this is an elective test that may not be covered by health insurance plans. Still, at approximately $375, I believe that the money spent for primary prevention will prove to be very cost-effective.

7. Where can I get the Ultrafast CT Scan performed?

Whether you are at high risk or just wish to receive a screening, call 1-800-469-HEART for the facility nearest you. Test results will be sent to your personal physician. For those without a private doctor, one on the staff of the attending hospital will be available for follow-up consultation.

Monitoring Your Heart During Exercise

A high-performance race car has a tachometer, a handy device next to the speedometer that registers just how hard the engine is working in a particular gear. As the engine reaches top speed in second gear, for example, the tachometer needle approaches the red line on the scale, and the gear is quickly shifted. As they compete, race car drivers are constantly checking the tachometer, making sure that they get within a hair's breadth of the red line without passing over it. This ensures them of maximum engine performance, without straining the motor.

For me, the human body is the race car and the heart is the high-performance engine. The heart-rate monitor is the equivalent of the tachometer. When you strap one around your chest, you now have the most precise gauge of exactly how hard your heart is working when you exercise. A simple three-part device, the monitor consists of a lightweight chest belt, a transmitter, and a watchlike receiver worn on the wrist. On the inner side of the chest belt are two electrodes that sense the heart's electrical signals, relaying that information to the transmitter. From there the data is continuously sent to the wrist monitor via an electromagnetic field. The monitor provides visual readouts such as heart rate and preselected target training zones for exercise.

The high-tech heart monitor is the single most important tool an exerciser can use today. By keeping within an age-related heart-rate boundary called your target heart rate, you can accurately and easily regulate the intensity and quality of your aerobic workout.

There are many companies making heart-rate monitors. However, I have been a longtime fan of the Polar Heart Rate Monitors (Polar Electro Inc., 99 Seaview Boulevard, Port Washington, NY 11050; tel. 1-800-227-1314) and recommend them to all of my patients. The monitors are used by world-class athletes who want precision in their training as well as by patients recovering from heart attacks who want to be sure that they don't push themselves too hard. A basic model called the Polar Excel sells for approximately $100.

Finding Your Target Heart Rate

Target heart rates are extremely effective in measuring not only your initial fitness levels, but also in monitoring your progress once you begin exercising on a regular basis. The best way to calculate your individual target heart rate is to use the mathematical age-adjusted maximum heart-rate formula. This entails subtracting your age from 220; the result is your theoretical maximum heart rate. As an equation it reads:

$$220 - \text{your age} = \text{age-adjusted maximum heart rate (MHR)}.$$

For instance, if you are forty years old, your age-adjusted maximum heart rate is:

$$220 - 40 = 180 \text{ beats per minute}$$

Once they have figured out their maximum heart rates, I like to have my patients exercising in one of two specific target heart zones. The moderate zone, which is 50 to 60 percent of your maximum rate, is used by men and women who are just starting an exercise program. By keeping their heart rates relatively low as they exercise, it ensures that they are able to go at an easy pace, with only slight breathlessness. Then, as their endurance levels improve, they can begin aerobic zone workouts.

The aerobic zone is for the patient who exercises regularly, and who can keep up a good pace for at least twenty to forty-five uninterrupted minutes.

The heart-rate zone you should exercise in is between 60 percent and 80 percent of your maximum heart rate.

The following table outlines the heart-rate ranges for different age groups, for both moderate and aerobic target heart zones. For example, if you are forty years old, the bulk of your exercise should fall somewhere within a range of 108 and 144 beats per minute. Look for your age category and check the ranges to find your moderate and aerobic target heart rates.

MHR	30 yrs.	40 yrs.	50 yrs.	60 yrs.	70 yrs.
80%	152	144	136	128	120
70%	133	126	119	112	105
60%	114	108	102	96	90
50%	95	90	85	80	75

What Can Be Done About "Silent" Heart Attacks?

Each year, about 1.5 million Americans will suffer a heart attack; approximately 350,000 of them will expire before reaching a hospital. Many of these men and women are victims of "silent ischemia," a heart attack that produces no typical "heart-related" symptoms such as mild indigestion.

Ischemia (pronounced iss-KEE-me-a), an acute or chronic shortage of oxygen to the heart, is nearly always caused by some form of atherosclerosis. Everyday stress, bursts of anger, and overexertion—whether it be work- or exercise-related—can place additional demands on the heart, producing ischemia that constricts the coronary artery even further, thereby blocking the blood flow to the heart. Patients with diabetes are also at increased risk of silent ischemia. In many cases, this narrowing produces a crushing pain called angina. This is the alert that warns a person to stop and calm down, seek help, or, if indicated, take medication. However, some studies have shown that ischemia without perceptible angina occurs roughly four times more often than ischemia with pain, and this silent killer is just as deadly.

No one is certain why inadequate blood flow to the heart produces the pain of angina in some patients and none in others. Some researchers point to a possible higher pain threshold for patients with silent ischemia. Regardless of the absence of pain, silent ischemia damages the heart muscle, greatly increasing the risk of heart attack and sudden death. Therefore, physicians are relying less on chest pains caused by angina to alert them to coronary artery disease, and instead look for other, more reliable, indicators of heart ailments.

One device used is the Holter monitor, which was developed to allow doctors to observe the action of a patient's heart at home or in the workplace. The idea behind this "ambulatory electrocardiogram" was very smart: It provides valuable information about changes in heart rhythm. Electrodes attach to the skin on the chest as the device records all heart rhythms on its computer chips during a continuous twenty-four-hour period. When the test is finished, the patient returns the recorder to his doctor for analysis.

Unfortunately, this monitor has its drawbacks. For one, the machine is cumbersome. For another, it rarely provides significant information about ischemia because its technology is limited to providing only a partial heart picture. For patients whose symptoms occur infrequently, the monitor—which is worn for only one day—will miss many of the faulty heart rhythm episodes. Studies have shown that at least two-thirds of this monitoring doesn't produce any positive information for the physician. Also, patients who wear the Holter monitor often change their daily habits, going out of their way to avoid stressful situations and trying to stay calm in order to "beat the machine."

The Age of the Cardiophone

One of the most exciting breakthroughs in detecting silent ischemia and cardiac arrhythmias is the Cardiophone, a miniature EKG machine developed by Globe-Tel that records cardiac episodes as they occur. This "event recorder" is usually used by a patient for a week or so; sometimes it is worn for a month or sometimes for as long as six months. The machine employs the latest technological advances, and offers the physician the best possible diagnostic capability by pinpointing both electrical and blood-flow problems of the heart. The monitor keeps a continuous record of the heart's electrical activities, picking up both heart arrhythmias as well as all signs of ischemia. This is especially important for those patients whose symptoms occur infrequently, and far away from their doctors' offices.

The Cardiophone records the reaction of a patient during his daily life, reflecting the heart's reaction to stress, anger, and problems. It also has the capacity to monitor and record blood pressure. Unlike the Holter monitor, which runs for a day, the lightweight Cardiophone can be worn for days. It is activated by pressing a red "record" button on the unit shortly after breakfast, before lunch, and again at dinner. Also, whenever a patient finds himself in a stressful situation, he is directed to activate the Cardiophone, thereby committing this vital heart information to the machine's memory. Another type of Cardiophone is a continuous memory loop—it runs constantly but does not permanently record information unless the button is pressed. When this happens, it records and stores the heartbeats for the thirty seconds prior to pressing the button, and then for the next thirty seconds as well.

As soon as is conveniently possible, the patient dials the toll-free Globe-Tel Diagnostics Receiving Center, which is staffed twenty-four hours a day, 365 days a year. After giving his name, Social Security number, and any significant health information to the operator (for example, "I was under a lot of stress," "I suddenly felt dizzy and weak," "I had a huge argument with my boss," "I felt a strange fluttering in my chest"), the patient's Cardiophone is placed to the phone mouthpiece and the "send" button is pressed. The machine then downloads all the vital heart information. Within a minute, the EKGs and pertinent health information are faxed to me.

Monitoring Your Heart in the Real World

The Cardiophone supplies doctors with clinical data from real-life situations, helping to assess heart health and allowing them to evaluate whether or not a patient has serious heart problems. Many times, patients have come to me complaining of possible heart problems, such as indigestion, palpitations, and light-headedness. Tests performed in the office will, many times, be inconclusive.

This is why the Cardiophone is so valuable: The lab goes with the patient. It helps to pinpoint whether symptoms are actually related to irregularities in heart rhythms, or ischemia, which is inadequate blood flow to the heart. Without having a patient in my office, I am given a window into his world. For example, I'm able to find out if chest pain is caused by atypical heart problems or by neurologic, metabolic, or pulmonary conditions. I can also determine if dizziness is caused by a pause in a heart rhythm or by some other problem.

Who Should Use the Cardiophone

Simple to use, the Cardiophone, which costs approximately $300 a month for continuous twenty-four-hour daily monitoring, can determine whether any suspicious symptoms are of cardiac origin. While it's uncommon to find considerable coronary artery disease in men under forty or in premenopausal women, cardiac risks do begin to increase with age. They start to rise as well in people with one or more of the seven major cardiac risk factors: a family history of heart disease, smoking, obesity, diabetes, hypertension, high cholesterol, and physical inactivity.

In general, I recommend Cardiophone screening for the following patients:

- men and women over forty with vague atypical cardiac symptoms
- men and women over forty who are planning on beginning a vigorous exercise program but have some fears they will have a heart attack
- men and women over forty involved in high-stress occupations or situations, especially those subject to excessive rage and anger
- men and women over fifty who have diabetes
- any patient with symptoms of heart palpitations, light-headedness, chest pain, shortness of breath, or dizziness
- patients whose "cardiac phobia" is limiting their lives
- post–heart attack, angioplasty, and bypass patients who are now at increased risk of suffering another cardiac event
- patients who are being monitored for blood pressure medications or heart rate

If evidence of insufficient blood flow to the heart or an abnormal cardiac rhythm is noted by the Cardiophone, a thorough cardiac evaluation is performed and early intervention is initiated.

If silent ischemia is indicated by the Cardiophone, treatment with prescription medication is often needed. For instance, beta-blocker drugs are used to reduce episodes of silent ischemia. Long-acting nitroglycerine also lessens the frequency and severity of this condition, as do calcium-channel blockers and antiarrhythmic drugs.

Many physicians are now using the Cardiophone—one of several cardiac event recorders currently available on the market—as a regular part of their preventive heart-care programs. To contact a doctor in your area who uses this new technology, write to or call Globe-Tel Diagnostics, Inc., 12700 Biscayne Blvd., North Miami Beach, FL 33181, 1-800-889-5383; or David Bluth, Granite Monitoring Services, Inc.; tel. 1-800-717-7543.

Female-Specific Heart Screening

Heart disease is the leading killer of women in this country, responsible for 34 percent of all female deaths—approximately 479,000 a year. What is particularly sobering is that more than half the women who die suddenly from heart attacks do not exhibit any prior evidence of cardiac disease.

I provide a preliminary cardiac profile for those female patients over the age of thirty-five participating in my Vitality Medicine program. After they fast for twelve hours, I employ a blood test that not only records their cholesterol and triglyceride levels, but four other coronary risk factors as well. They are:

- elevated lipoprotein (a), also known as Lp(a)
- increased fibrinogen
- elevated homocysteine
- decreased serum magnesium

The greater the presence of any of these four factors, the more likely the progression of atherosclerosis and its associated problems, namely heart attack and stroke. The earlier they are screened, the sooner they can be treated. Early detection can let doctors and patients know that a plan of action needs to be implemented, including making changes in diet, recommending the using of certain nutrients, and encouraging regular exercise.

Remember, any one result from a laboratory blood test, whether positive or negative, does not provide enough factual evidence to confirm or deny diagnosis. These tests must be viewed in the larger context of multiple risk factors and other diagnostic testing. When any of these risk factors is present, I repeat the blood tests again two to three months later. (**Note:** The tests must be specifically requested when blood is drawn and sent to a lab by your physician. Most large laboratories can perform them.) If abnormalities are confirmed, I then begin an aggressive cardioprotective program.

Lipoprotein(a)

Lipoprotein(a), commonly referred to as Lp(a), is now recognized as an independent risk factor for premature heart disease. In recent studies, it was found that elevated levels of Lp(a) predicted a twofold increase in the risk of developing heart disease by the age of fifty-five. This, researchers say, is about equal to the risk of having a high total cholesterol level.

Lp(a) is a fatty protein in the blood that is closely related to low-density lipoprotein, or LDL, also known as the "bad" cholesterol. Research seems to suggest that Lp(a) works by attaching to cholesterol, helping it travel through the bloodstream and depositing it on the arterial walls. There it forms fatty plaques or blood clots that block blood flow to the heart. Elevated Lp(a) also inhibits the normal dissolving of blood clots. Blood test results with levels above 30 mg/dl are considered to be abnormally high.

After menopause, Lp(a) levels usually begin to rise. However, this doesn't happen with women who take estrogen replacement, suggesting that estrogen plays a significant role in determining a woman's Lp(a) levels.

While there is currently no known way to lower high levels of Lp(a) other than using niacin, which often has unpleasant side effects, I use measurements of it to help construct an overall heart portrait of a patient. I find that abnormal test results serve as an effective tool to prompt patients to modify their coronary risk factors, which may include smoking, high blood cholesterol, high blood pressure, inactivity, and obesity.

Fibrinogen

A heart attack is not caused solely by atherosclerosis. Research now shows that the tendency for blood to clot, a process called thrombosis, is also a critical factor in whether or not a heart attack will occur.

Contrary to what scientists used to think, it's rare for plaque to completely block the flow of blood to the heart. It is now believed that small, unstable lesions covered by a fibrous cap actually cause a lot of the trouble. When the cap ruptures, the plaque starts to bleed, quickly triggering a clot to stanch the bleeding. It is this clotting that causes the heart attack.

Heart experts now realize that markers of risk are more directly related to a heightened hypercoagulability state in which the risk of developing blood clots is greatly increased. Fibrinogen is turning out to be one of those hypercoagulable factors.

A clotting precursor that has now been clearly identified as an independent risk factor for heart attack, fibrinogen is a protein that is converted to fibrin, the elastic filaments that form the framework of a clot. Some researchers believe that if your blood test shows high levels of this protein, then you have a higher risk of suffering a heart attack, as well as an increased risk of premature death. Others feel that a high level of fibrinogen is a greater danger component than elevated cholesterol. Only recently it has become known that:

- High levels of fibrinogen are more prevalent in women.
- Fibrinogen is more of a risk factor for women than for men.

Blood test results with levels above 350–400 mg/dl are considered to be dangerous.

Since smoking raises fibrinogen levels, the quickest way to lower its presence is to stop smoking. Also, you may be able to decrease fibrinogen levels by reducing your weight (if you need to) and eating a diet that is low in saturated fats while high in unsaturated ones. Taking a daily aspirin tablet of .81 mg can also impart anticlotting protection.

Homocysteine

A high level of the amino acid homocysteine is regarded as a serious risk factor of possible heart attack and stroke. Researchers aren't sure why, but elevated levels are nevertheless a more powerful predictor of these events in women than in men. Blood test results showing a range up to 16 micromoles per liter is considered safe. Anything above that number is considered abnormal.

Lack of B vitamins leads to homocysteine buildup. By modifying your diet and taking the right supplements, your homocysteine levels can drop to the safe range within a month or less.

The Homocysteine–Vitamin B Connection

An amino acid, homocysteine (homo-SIS-teen) is regarded by researchers to be as much a heart disease risk factor as smoking. Dr. Jacob Selhub, professor of nutrition at Tufts University, conducted a study of 1,041 subjects that linked folic acid deficiencies to increased clogged arteries and strokes in the elderly. He believes that if cholesterol accounts for half of all heart disease, then it is homocysteine that adds another possible 15 percent to the deadly equation.

The evidence from scientific research overwhelmingly indicates that low levels of B vitamins are a major contributor to heart disease. The reason is this: A deficiency of B vitamins—especially folic acid—permits the buildup of homocysteine.

Homocysteine develops when methionine, an amino acid needed for the formation of human proteins, breaks down. Eat a methionine-rich food, like eggs or hot dogs, and homocysteine levels will start to rise in your bloodstream. To keep homocysteine in check, your body relies on the help of three specific B vitamins: folic acid, B_6, and B_{12}. They reduce the levels of this amino acid, turning it back into methionine, and thereby reducing your risk of heart attack.

The Research

Some scientists, through their studies with baboons, pigs, and rabbits, believe that if your body is lacking any of these B vitamins, artery-clogging plaque starts to develop. Others believe that, like fibrinogen, homocysteine plays a role in hypercoagulability by prompting the construction of blood clots that eventually block arteries. This is accomplished when it builds up in the blood, causing the endothelial cells lining the coronary arteries to decrease their production of clot-dissolving substances. This activity increases the "stickiness" of the blood, which can lead to a heart attack. Finally, there are those who think that homocysteine, in combination with low-density lipoprotein, teams up to damage coronary arteries.

It is now estimated that a significant number of all heart attack patients, as well as a high percentage of stroke victims, have extremely high levels of homocysteine. There may be another contributing factor as well—age. Almost one-third of all patients over the age of sixty-seven involved in the Framingham Heart Study (an ongoing project begun in 1948 that has continuously followed 5,127 adults in Framingham, Massachusetts) had elevated homocysteine levels.

Other evidence implicating high levels of homocysteine as a heart risk continues to mount. A report in the *Journal of the American Medical Association* concluded that fourteen of seventeen heart studies found a correlation between elevated homocysteine levels and heart disease. When comparing blood levels of homocysteine and folic acid, twelve studies found that when the presence of homocysteine was elevated, that of folic acid was lowered. And nine studies on folic acid supplementation concurred that a decline in homocysteine levels is linked to taking extra vitamin B. Another *JAMA* study of more than five thousand subjects in the Nutrition Canada Survey supported these findings. It found that those Canadians with the lowest levels of folic acid blood levels had a 69 percent greater risk of death from coronary disease than those with the highest folic acid levels.

The healthy heart protectors, the B vitamins are easily accessible in both food and supplements. Increasing your intake of them, and folic acid in particular, should be a daily habit to reduce risk of heart disease.

Folic Acid

Also known as folate and folacin, folic acid helps protect against heart disease: *Researchers predict that just maintaining normal levels can prevent up to 50,000 deaths from heart disease each year.* Regrettably, it is estimated that only 12 percent of the U.S. adult population consumes the RDA (Recommended Daily Allowance) of folic acid daily, leaving the majority in a folate-deficient, and therefore heart-threatening, state.

By supplementing your diet with folic acid, whether by pill or by eating more folacin-fortified foods, you can reduce your blood levels of homocysteine to a safe range, and eliminate a very serious risk factor at the same time. The best strategies are outlined below and at the end of this chapter.

The Best Sources

Derived from the word *folium,* which means leaf, folic acid can be found in significant quantities in dark green leafy vegetables, especially spinach. Other sources, including dried beans (lentils, navy, kidney, and black beans are excellent suppliers), whole wheat, and citrus fruits contain high doses. One glass of orange juice will provide about 25 percent of your daily folic acid requirement. According to a new law, most enriched grain products, such as bread, flour, rice, and noodles, must be fortified with folic acid.

The Folic Acid Facts

To protect against a heart attack, *I recommend a daily minimum supplement of 400 mcg of folic acid to lower homocysteine to a safe level.* While fresh fruits and vegetables can supply all of your needs, taking a supplement will give you added insurance. Many common multiple vitamin supplements contain 400 mcg of folate; if you smoke you may need up to 600 mcg daily to get the same heart protection. Of course, the best heart protection is not to smoke at all.

Note: If you decide to take folic acid supplements, be sure to take a B_{12} supplement as well. Sometimes folic acid may mask signs of pernicious anemia, a condition caused by the body's inability to absorb vitamin B_{12}. If left unchecked, it can eventually lead to paralysis; alert your physician when you're taking folic acid.

Vitamin B_6

This water-soluble vitamin plays a large role in the metabolism of amino acids, which are used to create cells. Extremely sensitive, it is often in short supply in most people's diets, mainly because the body becomes less efficient in absorbing the vitamin. Women have to be especially careful to maintain their B_6 intake because they tend to consume fewer calories than men.

The Best Sources

Vitamin B_6 is found in chicken, fish, and pork, as well as in whole grains, legumes, bananas, raisins, sunflower seeds, and leafy green vegetables.

The Vitamin B_6 Facts

Low levels of vitamin B_6 are often found in heart-attack patients. Whether this deficiency is a cause or a result of the attack is not known. Also, inadequate levels of B_6 are thought to encourage the progress of atherosclerosis, increasing the risk of heart disease. Therefore, if you aren't eating enough of the foods that supply it, then *I recommend a daily B_6 supplement of 20 to 50 mg.*

Vitamin B_{12}

Vitamin B_{12} is necessary for the manufacture of red blood cells.

The Best Sources

Vitamin B_{12} is found only in animal products. Excellent sources are meat, fish, poultry, eggs, milk, and milk products.

The Vitamin B_{12} Facts

Most Americans supply themselves with enough B_{12} through their diet; in addition, they are able to store as much as 10 mg in their livers. However, strict vegetarians (vegans) who don't eat any animal products, as well as those who have a low intrinsic factor (the substance necessary to absorb vitamin B_{12} from foods), will need a supplement—orally, sublingually, or by injection—to meet the 3 mcg RDA. *I recommend 100 mcg of B_{12} daily.*

Magnesium

Deficiency of this mineral is more prevalent in women than in men, and is thus more predictive of coronary disease in women. In the heart, it prevents spasms of coronary arteries and abnormal heart rhythms that can lead to sudden death. It also helps to deter the formation of blood clots that plug arteries and trigger heart attacks by inhibiting the release of substances that make blood platelets stickier and more apt to form clots.

Blood test results showing 2 mg/dl of magnesium are considered normal. Anything lower is an indicator of deficiency and needs to be watched closely by your physician. Diminished levels are indicators for possible heart disease.

The Research

During the past ten years, magnesium has received considerable attention in heart research. It plays a critical role in the functioning of over three hundred of the body's enzymes (which are chemicals that regulate bodily functions). It also assists in the maintenance of nerve and muscle cells, as well as the contraction of muscles. Studies now suggest that magnesium deficiencies have a definite effect on heart function. Some of the findings have shown that:

- People with high blood pressure often have below-average magnesium levels.
- Heart patients with congestive heart failure and magnesium deficiencies were more likely to have irregular heartbeats and to die within a year when compared to patients with normal magnesium levels.
- Magnesium insufficiencies can lead to:
    1. constriction of blood vessels;
    2. decrease in high-density lipoprotein cholesterol (the "good" kind);
    3. high blood pressure;
    4. increase in low-density lipoprotein cholesterol;
    5. tachyarrhythmia (rapid heart beat).

A 1995 survey found that almost three of four adults fall short of the daily allowance for magnesium. More than half consume less than three-quarters of the recommended amount. Researchers speculate that when quantities of magnesium in the body are insufficient, cell membranes become more prone to free-radical attacks and their subsequent damage.

The Best Sources

Wheat germ, wheat bran, nuts, soybeans, corn, and dark leafy vegetables are all good sources of magnesium. However, many people don't eat these foods in sufficient quantities, which means they're probably not getting enough daily magnesium.

The Magnesium Facts

People at high risk for deficiency include heavy drinkers, hypertension patients on diuretics, and insulin-dependent diabetics. The RDA for magnesium is 350 mg for males, 280 mg for females. *I recommend a daily intake of three 200 mg pills of magnesium chloride.* If you have already had a heart attack, consult with your physician before taking any magnesium supplements.

When Cardiovascular Risks Coincide with Risk for Osteoporosis

When women are in the postmenopausal years, the natural drop in levels of the hormone estrogen leaves them vulnerable to the dual problems of heart disease and osteoporosis. This double health problem is not uncommon. Unfortunately, it's one that won't have more definitive solutions until at least 2007, the year when the Women's Health Initiative is completed. This fifteen-year study—the largest study of women's health ever undertaken in the United States—will help determine, among other things, the overall risk of long-term hormone therapy to the heart and bones. However, by intervening early with a comprehensive risk-reduction plan, a woman has a good chance to prevent and halt the progress of both diseases.

Hormone replacement therapy, or HRT, a combination of estrogen and another hormone called progestin, is a first line of defense that all women should consider. Studies have shown that long-term HRT can protect against heart disease and the bone loss of osteoporosis.

Decisions for the Heart

Working together with her physician, a woman should weigh the benefits and risks of long-term hormone use and make her decision. HRT is certainly not for every woman. Factored into each woman's decision is the family history of heart disease, osteoporosis, and cancer, as well as risk factors such as smoking, cholesterol levels, and bone density.

The HRT Effect

Heart disease kills more women than all cancers combined, and a woman's chances of dying from heart disease are ten times greater than dying from breast cancer. Several studies suggest that HRT can cut the risk of heart disease in half. If your risk of heart disease is high due to your family history, and you also have a low risk of breast cancer, then you're a good candidate for HRT.

The HRT Facts

Physicians typically prescribe HRT combining estrogen and progestin. Estrogen can be taken by injection, in pill form, as a vaginal cream, or as a time-release patch. Progestin is typically taken in pill form. Your physician will work out a HRT schedule with you based on your symptoms. You may take estrogen for a certain number of days, then take progestin along with estrogen for a certain number of days, and then stop one or both of the medications for a period of time. This schedule is repeated every month and often causes monthly bleeding similar to a menstrual period. Other possible side effects of HRT can include fluid retention, weight gain, and headaches. However, an alternative dosing schedule is to prescribe daily HRT and this usually stops regular monthly bleeding.

To be effective, HRT has to be taken long-term. Researchers are still investigating the full implications of HRT use of ten years or more. Again, talk over your options with your physician.

Statin Medications

Along with improving her diet and increasing her level of physical activity, a woman now has other solutions to the heart-bone dilemma if high cholesterol is a problem. In addition to niacin, which is available over the counter, and bile acid–binding resins (Colestid and Questran), prescription drugs that can lower LDL cholesterol by as much as 20 percent, a brand-new class of effective cholesterol-lowering drugs called **statins** has been found to offer exceptional heart protection.

The Statin Effect

Statin medications can lower cholesterol and help prevent the formation and progression of atherosclerosis. The groundbreaking West of Scotland Study (1995) dramatically showed that by using pravastatin (Pravachol, the brand name), heart disease can effectively be prevented by lowering cholesterol. The Scottish study evaluated over 6,000 men aged forty-five to sixty-four who had no history of heart disease and followed them for five years. At the start of the study, their total cholesterol levels ranged from 250 to 295 mg/dl, with LDL levels ranging from 150 to a high of 232 mg/dl.

When compared to a placebo group, the men who were given pravastatin for the duration of the study had reduced their cholesterol by 20 percent, with a 26 percent drop in LDL cholesterol. Also, levels of HDL ("good") cholesterol rose by 5 percent. While this study only looked at the effects of pravastatin on men, many experts now believe that the same heart-protective benefits of the medication can reasonably be expected for women as well.

The Statin Facts

Pravastatin is one of a group of several statin medications; the others are lovastatin (Mevacor), simvastatin (Zocor), fluvastatin (Lescol), and atorvastatin (Lipitor), which received FDA approval in December 1996. Each requires a specific dose to lower cholesterol. The decision as to which of these statin drugs is used depends on the degree of cholesterol elevation and an individual's response to the medication. These prescription drugs are taken daily in 10 to 20 mg doses and help reduce cholesterol by interfering with its production in the liver and increasing the removal of LDL from the blood. A month's supply of the drugs costs approximately $120. *They have to be taken long-term in order to keep cholesterol levels down.*

As with any medication, some people may have adverse reactions to the statin drugs, including mild gastrointestinal disturbances, muscle pain, or headache. Also, a lupus-like syndrome (an inflammatory disorder that affects many body parts) has been reported in some patients using lovastatin and pravastatin.

The Osteoporosis Decisions

Osteoporosis, which means "porous bones," has its own set of special considerations, particularly because many women now live a quarter to a third of their lives after menopause. Osteoporosis occurs naturally with age, but because the female hormone estrogen helps maintain bone strength, women are more prone to develop this ailment once estrogen levels are dramatically reduced during the first few years following menopause. It's now estimated that a minimum of 10 percent of women over the age of fifty suffer from bone loss severe enough to cause fracture of the hip, spine, and long bones of the arm and leg.

While there is currently no cure for the bone fragility brought on by osteoporosis, nor can it be totally prevented, fortunately it can be delayed and its severity lessened with several treatment options designed to prevent further bone loss. In addition to a calcium-rich diet and weight-bearing exercise, HRT is one of the major preventive choices a woman should consider. This effective hormone therapy helps prevent osteoporosis as well as protect against heart disease.

Although there is a preponderance of medical evidence showing that HRT prevents the accelerated bone loss that comes with menopause—there is also a consistently noted 30 to 50 percent drop in hip, wrist, and spine fractures in women who use HRT for five years—HRT is not appropriate for everyone because it may also increase the risk of uterine and breast cancer for some women. Therefore, the patient, along with her physician, must carefully weigh her own situation along with all the risks and benefits of HRT.

The use of **calcitonin,** a naturally occurring hormone that's strictly involved in the metabolism of bone and calcium regulation, is a possible treatment option for women who cannot or choose not to use the sex hormone–based HRT for halting osteoporosis. Calcitonin, which is available as a nasal spray, helps prevent further bone loss by slowing down the bone removal process.

Fosamax

If you cannot or choose not to use HRT and don't want to use calcitonin, a new nonhormonal medication for osteoporosis called **Fosamax** (alendronate) can also be considered to help remedy the bone-thinning problems you may have. This medication (approved by the FDA in 1995) has been found to increase bone mass by as much as 8 percent and reduce fractures by as much as 40 percent. To avoid any side effects, Fosamax must be taken according to label directions.

Fosamax Facts

This medication, which costs approximately $50 per month, has to be taken daily for the long term. One 10 mg tablet is taken on an empty stomach with plenty of water immediately upon awakening. The patient should not lie down, take other medications, eat, or drink anything but plain water for at least thirty minutes. Patients who have esophagus abnormalities should not be using this medication. The drug may have minor side effects that include heartburn, gas, nausea, and abdominal pain. To date, there have been no studies completed comparing its efficacy with HRT use, nor are there any completed studies examining the combined use of HRT *and* Fosamax. For the present time, Fosamax cannot be recommended for use in conjunction with HRT.

While Fosamax is currently only approved for osteoporosis treatment, the FDA is expected soon to okay its use as an *osteoporosis preventive medication,* taken long term on a daily basis by healthy women in a 5 mg dose.

DEXA: Testing for Osteoporosis

The best way to gauge your risk for osteoporosis is to have your bone mass measured. Loss of bone in women can begin as early as thirty-five, and typically without any symptoms. Therefore, as a preventive measure, a woman should know her current bone density status. **Bone density,** the amount of bone mass, can now be quickly and effectively measured and the risk of bone fracture assessed with a readily available test called DEXA (dual X-ray absorptiometry). A good time for a woman to be tested is when she reaches menopause, but if you are concerned about your bone status, it's never too late to be checked out.

After a simple five- to twenty-minute X-ray of your hip and/or spine, the results are compared to a standard for your age and body size. Based on these results, your physician can then make preventive recommendations, which can include starting HRT or Fosamax, in addition to increasing daily calcium consumption and regular weight-bearing exercise. A follow-up DEXA, within one to two years, is recommended to determine the effectiveness of your treatment.

Determining the Best Health Strategy

1. **Smoking**
   Aim: Complete cessation.
   Recommendation: Seek out counseling, begin nicotine replacement therapy, or join a smoking-cessation program.

2. Cholesterol

Aim: Lower LDL cholesterol to under 100 mg/dl, raise HDL levels to above 50 mg/dl, and lower triglyceride levels to below 100 mg/dl.

Recommendations:

a. Start a low-fat eating plan that stresses an intake of less than 30 percent fat.

b. Have your physician perform a fasting lipid panel test that checks levels of cholesterol, HDL cholesterol, LDL cholesterol, and triglycerides.

c. After initiating your low-fat eating plan and regular exercise, repeat the test in one to three months. Based on these test results, here are your options:

- If your HDL level is less than 35 mg/dl, *talk with your physician* about a low-fat eating plan and starting a course of exercise. Also, *talk to your physician* about the possible use of niacin to raise your HDL level.

- If your LDL level is below 100 mg/dl, continue with your current diet and exercise plan.

- If your LDL level is between 100 and 130 mg/dl and you have coronary artery disease (CAD), *talk with your physician* about taking statin medication or alternative drugs such as niacin and resins. If you do not have CAD and are at otherwise low risk for CAD (no other risk factors), *talk to your physician* about measures necessary to lower it to 100 mg/dl or less.

- If your LDL level is above 130 mg/dl, *seriously consider* using statin medication to reduce your level, especially if you have other CAD risk factors.

- If your triglyceride level is above 175 mg/dl but less than 200 mg/dl, *no medications are necessary.* Continue with your diet and exercise and try to lower triglycerides to 100 mg/dl or below.

- If your triglyceride level is between 200 and 400, *seriously consider* a course of statin drugs or niacin.

- If your triglyceride level is above 400 mg/dl,

seriously consider the combination of statin medication and niacin.

3. **Osteoporosis**
   Aim: To prevent the progression of osteoporosis.
   Recommendations:
   a. Begin a calcium-rich eating plan, increasing your daily intake of calcium to 1,000 mg if you're taking HRT, 1,500 mg if you're not. If your diet is deficient, take a calcium carbonate supplement daily to maintain calcium intake.
   b. Assess your bone density with a DEXA test. If your DEXA is normal, continue with your calcium-rich diet and regular exercise. If your DEXA is abnormal:
      • Discuss *long-term* HRT with your physician. This must be individualized according to your personal health risks.
      • Discuss *long-term* Fosamax use with your physician.
      • Discuss *long-term* calcitonin use with your physician.

4. **Physical activity**
   Aim: Thirty minutes three times per week.
   Recommendations:
   a. Talk with your physician to assess your physical risks before beginning a regular exercise program.
   b. Aim for three thirty-minute weight-bearing workouts per week. Walking, jogging, aerobics, stairclimbing, and weight training are excellent choices.
   c. If osteoporosis is advanced, ask your physician for a recommendation for a physical therapist who can design an exercise program to strengthen your hips and back.

5. **Weight**
   Aim: To keep within healthy weight and body-fat levels for your age and height.
   Recommendations:
   a. Start a low-fat eating plan.
   b. Begin a regular exercise program, as outlined above.

   c. If obese, discuss the possible use of weight-loss
      medication (phentermine, fenfluramine, dexfenflu-
      ramine) with your physician.
6. **Estrogen**
   Aim: To reduce risk of atherosclerotic heart disease and
     osteoporosis, as well as any menopausal symptoms of
     vaginal atrophy and dryness, hot flashes, and mood
     changes.
   Recommendation: Discuss the pros and cons of *long-
   term* HRT with your physician.

How to S.A.V.E. Your Heart

Stress is a factor all of us live with. But how we do—or
don't—deal with it can injure our hearts. Unchecked, it can
lead to early heart disease.

Researchers at Duke University are now actively exploring how the heart and mind interact in response to everyday stress. They think the connection between the two may
be so strong that testing for mental stress will be used to
predict the risk of heart attack in certain people. In fact,
they believe that in five years or so this testing may actually become part of a doctor's routine exam.

In their recent study published in the *Journal of the
American Medical Association,* the Duke scientists gave
five special mental-stress tests to 126 subjects. These mental exercises mimicked some of the everyday stresses all of
us encounter. Next, the results were processed, and compared to those who took standard physical exercise stress
tests. The outcome of the mental tests was intriguing:

*When compared to patients who exhibited low levels of
mental stress during testing, those patients who displayed
stress-related cardiac changes during testing were almost
three times more likely to have a heart attack, or some other
cardiac event, in the ensuing months.*

Dr. Wei Jiang, a cardiologist and lead author of the Duke
study, believes that the particular lifestyle of Americans
puts us at an elevated risk for cardiac events: "Based on
our studies of patients with coronary artery disease, I can

theoretically say that stress has a major impact on the development of coronary artery disease in healthy people."

By not properly dealing with daily stressors and lessening their impact, two physical reactions take place:

• As blood pressure rises, patches of endothelial cells, which line the coronary arteries, begin to erode. This is due to the rapidly swirling currents of blood rushing through the arteries.

• Fats, which are held in reserve for emergencies, pour into the bloodstream and head to the damaged arterial walls. Over time, these fats will create arteriosclerotic plaques that can block the flow of blood to the heart and eventually lead to a heart attack.

The S.A.V.E. Technique

Ridding our lives of stress is an impossibility; however, the importance we give it and the way we handle it can make an enormous difference in the basic health of our heart. My solution was to develop the S.A.V.E. technique, and use it as part of my Vitality Medicine program for stress reduction—and therefore heart disease prevention. It is designed as a self-help aid for those people who are continually subjected to stress on the job or at home.

A progressive, four-step program that will help you to deter or reduce everyday stress, S.A.V.E. consists of:

Step 1: Stop in your tracks. The programmed response to stress can be undermined if you simply stop and think about what you are doing. Most people realize they are in the midst of a stress-filled situation, but all too often choose to ignore their own intuition. Instead, they make the critical mistake of thinking that if they confront the issue, person, or people triggering their response, the situation will be resolved.

At the onset of stress, I advise my patients to simply take several deep breaths or just count to ten slowly. Sometimes that is all that is needed to get over the stress and turn off the flow of adrenaline and cortisol that can harm your heart. In some situations, distancing yourself physically will provide the much-needed time to think of an alternative means of handling the problem in a less stressful way. At the very least, it will allow you to:

Step 2: Assess the situation carefully, and decide whether it actually merits further attention. Prioritize, and take into account time constraints as well as the bigger picture. This way, you can develop an effective plan of action that acknowledges, as well as takes into consideration, both your limitations and vulnerabilities.

If your current stress situation demands further action, you need to think rationally about what your next step needs to be. It will help if you ask yourself these five questions:

1. Am I willing to accept the stress-inducing terms of my current situation?
2. If I am, why?
3. How important is it that this be done right now?
4. What is the worst thing that can happen to me if I don't accept the terms of the situation?
5. Is there a way to modify the terms so that they are more compatible to my own particular style, thereby reducing the stressors that are creating tension?

After answering these questions as honestly as possible, you are ready to:

Step 3: Visualize yourself handling this situation differently. Give yourself the opportunity to view yourself without time constraints, calmly making rational decisions from a variety of viable options within your control. Now you can anticipate any possible difficulties and mentally plan how you will alter their effects. The mind is a very powerful tool that you can tap into; by mentally rehearsing your strategy, you can circumvent stressful situations because you can anticipate pitfalls and minefields before they happen.

To begin, close your eyes and visualize yourself moving effortlessly through each stage of the problem. Note how comfortable and experienced you are: You can handle any situation with calm and expertise, no matter how difficult the challenge.

Your confidence secure, you now have the momentum to work your way through each step of the obstacle successfully, making progress without a hitch. This enables you to:

Step 4: Enact your plan. Now you are ready, willing, and able to implement your stress solutions. Your path is clear:

- Think about your "enactment plan" of short- and long-term goals.
- Have a clear, focused vision that is understandable to everyone involved in the situation.
- Break down your plan into manageable segments.
- Consult, if you can, with friends and experts for advice and listen to their opinions.
- Put your plan into action.
- Do the best you can under the circumstances—and accept the outcome.

Congratulate yourself on a job well done and be aware of what you have achieved in the least stressful way. Once you see how well S.A.V.E. works, you will want to use it again until it becomes your habitual response to stress-filled situations.

Ensuring Your Heart's Health

Helping our hearts to maintain their health and warding off the potential for life-threatening disease is simpler than you thought. Vitamins B, C, and E, the antioxidants coenzyme Q10 (see page 196) and Pycnogenol, the mineral magnesium, and as common a drug as aspirin have been medically proven to offer maximum heart protection. Taking them is not only a recommendation; it is a necessity for those who want to keep their hearts beating steadily and strongly now and for years to come. They are an integral part of my Vitality Medicine program.

Increase Your Vitamin C Intake

Vitamin C does much more than just protect you from the ravages of the common cold. Researchers have long pointed out the critical role that this antioxidant vitamin plays in the prevention of atherosclerosis, thereby helping the heart. It does so by:

- increasing the permeability as well as the strength of capillaries
- inhibiting blood clotting
- reducing both cholesterol and fat levels
- repairing red blood cells

The Research

The current RDA for vitamin C is 60 mg, and may be justified for disease prevention. Unfortunately, it is far from optimal for a healthy life. This was proved in a recently released study from the National Institutes of Health (NIH), which delved into the varying vitamin C dosages to determine which was the most effective. The men taking part in the study were first fed a diet deficient in vitamin C. Then they were given vitamin C sequentially in seven specific dosages: 30, 60, 200, 400, 1,000, and 2,500 mg. The results showed that:

- With 30 mg the subjects became irritable and fatigued from lack of the vitamin.
- With 200 mg the blood plasma levels were almost totally saturated with vitamin C.
- At 1,000 and 2,500 mg the blood plasma was completely saturated but at the higher dosage less vitamin C was absorbed from the intestines and more was eliminated in the urine. Also, the urine contained oxalate and urate, two breakdown products of vitamin C that contribute to the formation of kidney stones.

The NIH researchers now believe that an intake of vitamin C below 1,000 mg a day is safe (it doesn't cause diarrhea) but that dosages above 400 mg have "no evident value."

The Best Sources

Citrus fruits, like oranges, grapefruits, and tangerines, are superior sources of vitamin C. It is also present in most fruits and vegetables, including melons, strawberries, red peppers, dark green leafy vegetables, potatoes, and tomatoes.

The Vitamin C Facts

For optimal levels of vitamin C, *I now recommend at least 200 mg of vitamin C daily for maximal antioxidant power and heart disease protection.* While food is the best source of vitamin C, if you are like most of your fellow Americans who do not eat the recommended five servings a day of fruits and vegetables (the U.S. average intake is only three), then a supplement is definitely in order.

Increase Your Vitamin E Intake

A powerful antioxidant that protects against heart disease by preventing the oxidation of LDL cholesterol that builds up and forms plaque on arterial walls, vitamin E also helps to reduce the clotting ability of the blood.

The Research

In the Cambridge Heart Antioxidant Study, one thousand men and women with heart disease were given a placebo, while another one thousand test subjects took vitamin E. For two years, five hundred of them took 800 IU (International Units, each of which contains almost 1 mg) daily while the other five hundred downed 400 IU daily for one year. Researchers noted a significant factor in the groups receiving vitamin E:

- After six months, the risk of heart attack dropped by nearly 80 percent.
- After eighteen months, both groups receiving vitamin E had a quarter of the number of heart attacks as the placebo group.

A recent study from the University of Texas Southwestern Medical Center in Dallas divided forty-eight men into six random groups. They were assigned to receive either a placebo or vitamin E capsules in dosages of 60, 200, 400, 800, and 1,200 IU daily for eight weeks. Blood cholesterol levels were checked before and after the study. Those men who took 400 IU of vitamin E had significantly less oxidation of LDLs than any other group. This means that the minimum amount of vitamin E necessary to keep LDL cholesterol from sticking to coronary artery walls is 400 IU.

The Best Sources

Getting adequate quantities of vitamin E that offer heart protection from food is often a problem. Most of my patients who adhere to low-fat diets have difficulty taking in even the minimum amount of the vitamin (8 IU for men and 10 IU for women). This is because vitamin E is found primarily in high-fat foods such as nuts, seeds, vegetable oils, and mayonnaise (it is present in dark, leafy vegetables as well). Therefore, the best way to ensure that they are getting enough daily vitamin E is through a supplement.

The Vitamin E Facts

Although the RDA is 8 to 10 IU, which is adequate for dietary deficiencies, *I recommend 400 IU daily for heart protection.*

Note: Consult with your physician first before beginning vitamin E supplementation if you have any type of bleeding disorder or if you are taking any kind of anticoagulant medication. There is a very small risk that high doses of vitamin E may raise your risk of hemorrhagic stroke, in which bleeding occurs in the brain.

A Final Word About Vitamins
C and E

The mighty antioxidant power of vitamins C and E in heart disease prevention is beyond dispute. A nine-year study of 11,000 men and women over the age of sixty-seven was reported in the *American Journal of Clinical Nutrition* in 1996. The researchers compared their subjects with people who did not use either vitamin C or E supplements. They found that:

- Subjects who took vitamin E supplements had 34 percent fewer deaths from any cause than those who took none.
- Subjects who took both vitamin C and E supplements separately on a regular basis (not in a multivitamin) had a 40 percent reduced risk of dying from any cause.
- Subjects who used either vitamin C or E had a 50 percent reduced risk of dying of heart disease.

While scientists are just beginning to understand how these nutrients work within a body, it is now becoming quite obvious that a daily high intake of them, either from food or supplements, plays a major protective role against heart disease.

Increase Your Intake of
Coenzyme Q10

Along with Pycnogenol (see Chapter 5), coenzyme Q10 (CoQ10) is an antioxidant nutrient that is being hailed for its capacity to help prevent and combat heart disease.

CoQ10 is a vital factor for enzymes involved in energy metabolism in all human cells. First called ubiquinone because it is so prevalent in the human body, it is present in each cell. Since CoQ10 is critical in the conversion of food to energy, it is found more abundantly in some tissue cells than in others. Concentrations of the enzyme are particularly high in the heart, researchers believe, since that organ requires an enormous amount of energy to pump blood throughout the body.

CoQ10 was first isolated in 1957 by Dr. Frederick Crane, a biology professor at the University of Wisconsin, who extracted it from cattle heart mitochondria. However, Japanese scientists eventually did most of the work involved in synthesizing and developing CoQ10 into supplement form. In 1974, the government of Japan approved the use of CoQ10; now as many as fifteen million Japanese take it daily as a nutritional supplement or as medication for heart disease.

Just how CoQ10 works is still not fully understood. Scientists do know, from animal studies, that it acts as an antioxidant that prevents free radicals, which are viewed as major contributors to heart disease, from attacking and damaging cardiac cells. CoQ10 does this by stabilizing cell membranes, keeping them from being destroyed.

The Research

Various studies have shown that as we age, the loss of CoQ10 in the heart muscle is considerable. The CoQ10 levels of some heart patients are as much as 75 percent lower than those of healthy patients. In fact, these diminished levels may be strong indicators of impending death from heart disease. A small Swedish study of ninety-four hospital patients fifty years old and up found that those who died within six months had considerably lower CoQ10 levels than the survivors.

Increasing CoQ10 levels, however, seems to have a pronounced positive effect on heart health. Research carried out by Karl Folkers, Ph.D., the director of the Institute for Biomedical Research at the University of Texas at Austin, bears this out. In Folker's study, 126 patients with cardiomyopathy, a serious degeneration of the heart muscle that often leaves patients in need of a heart transplant, were followed. Before taking CoQ10, the yearly death rate from this debilitating cardiac disease ranged from 35 percent to 65 percent. However, after patients started taking CoQ10, death rates dropped and evened off at 9 percent. Five years later, death rates from all causes was 48 percent—but only one-third were due to cardiac causes.

In addition to offering heart protection, CoQ10 has been found to impart a dramatic effect on elevated blood pressure. In a study conducted by cardiologist Peter Langsjoen, along with researchers at the University of Texas at Austin, 109 patients with hypertension were given 225 mg of CoQ10 every day. This amount significantly lowered the blood pressure in ninety-two of the test subjects. While it had no effect on sixteen of the patients, the condition of only one worsened.

The patients whose conditions were improved by taking CoQ10—and they rallied within three to four months of daily use—had lower blood pressure. Their systolic (upper number reading) pressure was down, from an average of 159 to 147, as was their diastolic (lower number reading) pressure, from an average of 94 to 85. Because of the CoQ10 supplementation, more than forty of the patients were able to stop taking one or more of their hypertension medications, while another twenty began using CoQ10 alone to manage their hypertension.

The Best Sources

CoQ10 is found, in small quantities, in seafood, eggs, and in all fruits and vegetables. The average person consumes approximately 5 mg of CoQ10 daily, a quantity considered by many experts to be too low to meet the needs of the body, especially after the age of fifty. As we age, CoQ10 levels begin to drop; by the time we reach middle age, many of us have barely 20 percent of the CoQ10 levels we had in our twenties. This dropoff may be due to free-radical activity in the mitochondria, the furnaces of the cells. As we know, free radicals damage our cells, leading to heart disease and other chronic ailments.

The CoQ10 Facts

Since most people in their forties and fifties have lowered CoQ10 levels and don't take in enough in their daily diet, supplementation is advised. *For heart protection, I recom-*

mend 30 mg of CoQ10 daily. If you already have heart disease, or have risk factors for it, take 60 to 100 mg daily. It is available in all health food stores. I suggest taking the softgel that is mixed with oil; it is more easily absorbed than the dry tablets.

Increase Your Intake of Aspirin

One of the world's most popular drugs, aspirin may turn out to be the most cost-effective heart medication available for both men and women. Taken on a regular basis, aspirin inhibits the formation of blood clots, the fine, gelatin-like globs that can quickly block the vital arteries that supply the heart with blood.

The Research

Convincing and powerful evidence for aspirin's amazing heart-protecting qualities first surfaced in 1988. That was when the results of the Physicians' Health Study were first announced. In that study, 11,000 doctors who had taken a standard 325 mg aspirin tablet every other day for the previous five years were shown to have a very considerable 44 percent lower rate of heart attacks when compared to another group of 11,000 who took a placebo.

While this research, and many other studies, have only been conducted on men, a larger study of 40,000 female health care workers is now being conducted by Harvard scientists to test the effectiveness of aspirin in the prevention of heart disease; results should be available in a few years. Since there is no evidence that aspirin is harmful and it appears to be helpful, I currently recommend aspirin to my female patients as well.

The Aspirin Facts

Since aspirin is such a powerful thrombolytic agent (from the Greek words *thrombus,* meaning clot, and *lysis,* to dissolve), *I now recommend a standard daily enteric-coated low-dose 81 mg (baby) aspirin for all of my healthy patients over fifty. I also recommend it for all patients who have hypertension, high blood cholesterol, or present any heart disease risk factor.*

As with all medications, consult with your physician first before beginning the aspirin regimen. Aspirin, in combination with certain medications you may already be taking, may cause problems.

SUMMARY OF HEART PROTECTIVE SOURCES AND RECOMMENDATIONS

Heart Protector	Primary Food Source	Daily Recommendation
Folic Acid	Green leafy vegetables, citrus fruits	400 mcg
Vitamin B$_6$	Chicken, fish, pork, whole grains, legumes, fruits, and green leafy vegetables	20 to 50 mg
Vitamin B$_{12}$	Meat, fish, eggs, poultry, milk products	100 mcg
Vitamin C	Citrus fruits, cantaloupe, strawberries, tomatoes, potatoes, red peppers, dark green leafy vegetables	200 mg
Vitamin E	Whole grains, wheat germ, nuts, vegetable oils, and dark green leafy vegetables	400 IU
Coenzyme Q10	Seafood, eggs, fruits, and vegetables	30 mg; 60 to 100 mg with heart disease
Pycnogenol	Not applicable	1.5 mg per lb. body weight for 10 days; .75 mg per lb. body weight thereafter
Magnesium	Wheat germ, wheat bran, nuts, soybeans, corn, and dark leafy vegetables	200 mg twice daily
Aspirin	Not applicable	One .81 mg enteric-coated baby aspirin for patients over 50

Note: A healthy diet, exercise, and cardioprotective doses of vitamins B, C, and E are recommended for everyone. As is the case with all aspects of Vitality Medicine, the program should be individually tailored for each person.

Certain vitamins do double duty, protecting not only the heart but assisting in memory enhancement as well. Remember, if you take a vitamin such as B_6 for added heart protection, you'll be getting the memory-boosting power from the vitamin as well, so be sure not to double dose by duplicating that amount when following other Vitality Medicine recommendations. In all cases, consult your physician for the best way to individualize your program.

Primary Prevention: Your Number-One Goal

As you by now have come to understand, the basis of my heart protection program is to prevent surprises and leave you with no regrets. I am a big proponent of primary prevention, and I do everything in my power to improve a patient's state of health. There is currently a tremendous amount of medical evidence that provides grounds for improving heart health and vitality. By utilizing new technology, techniques, and medications, you and I can become equal participants in the practice of Vitality Medicine.

7

Endurance Unlimited

Most of the men and women I see as patients are high-achievers, people who begin their days at a running start and don't stop until late in the evening. This lifestyle can be a choice, a necessity, or both. Whatever the reasons, the demands are unrelenting, though the rewards great. Slowing down isn't an option when the need to compete, nurture, and succeed are daily challenges.

If there is one enemy common to these driven people, regardless of age, it is fatigue. Endurance is the force they need to perform, sustaining their energy and focus. It is an essential strength and they cannot afford to lose it.

If I had to choose the most important component of my Vitality Medicine program, it would be the ability to enhance and maintain endurance. With increased stamina, my patients feel empowered. They have a keen advantage over their opponents: the ability to be in control of themselves and any tough situations that come their way. Without it, they are doomed to winding down, losing their edge, falling behind. With it, they have optimal physical and mental power, which translates seamlessly to peak performance.

Good Health Doesn't Guarantee Endurance

Being disease-free is, of course, a desirable state. Determined as much by luck and genetics as by diet and exercise, good health is something all of us want. But being disease-free is not enough if you want to live your life fully and effectively. In fact, the MacArthur Foundation's study of aging in America has found that lifestyle overrides genetics. Living at "full throttle"—certainly the breakneck pace of millions of men and women—in fact *extends* longevity. This makes endurance all the more important, because, it seems, the harder you live your life, the longer you are going to live. My power-building component of Vitality Medicine provides the necessary tools to defeat fatigue and harness energy.

This was the case with Len, a fifty-two-year-old corporate attorney who had been blessed with good health his entire life. He couldn't remember the last time he had had a cold. So it was with considerable concern that he came to see me, complaining that he was tired so frequently that both his business life and private life were being affected.

"I don't know what's wrong with me," he said. "I don't feel any pain. Nothing 'hurts' me. But I feel exhausted all the time—and it's bothering me a lot. I still use the treadmill at the gym three times a week but it doesn't seem to make any difference. My work is slowing down and my personal life is on hold. Am I sick?"

Whenever a patient comes to me with exhaustion as the primary symptom the first thing I do is try to rule out illness. Once we established that Len was, indeed, as healthy and disease-free as ever, I gave him a MicroFit Endurance Evaluation. Composed of seven factors, the evaluation gives a clear indication of why endurance is low, and how it can be improved upon. The factors, which will be discussed in detail later in this chapter, are: percentage of body fat, biceps strength, flexibility, resting heart rate, systolic blood pressure, diastolic blood pressure, and aerobic endurance.

In Len's case, we found that his percentage of body fat

was too high, his blood pressure readings and resting heart rate were acceptable for his age, but his muscular strength and flexibility fell into the unfit level. Even though he was aerobically fit, due to his regular use of the treadmill, his strength and overall endurance were less than optimal.

My recommendation for Len was weight training, which could help him to:

- eliminate fatigue
- improve glucose utilization
- strengthen bones, thereby staving off the onset of osteoporosis by increasing bone density
- enhance his sex life by decreasing fat levels and raising testosterone levels
- speed up metabolism, allowing him to control weight gain

And, of course, he would be able to make his already fit body look even better.

Everyone who needs to build endurance will benefit by weight training. Implementing a regular program is the best way for you to:

- lower blood pressure
- pare away body fat around the waist and hips and lose extra pounds
- support the more than two hundred bones in the body and thereby achieve better posture
- prevent injuries
- develop a contoured body
- stop *sarcopenia,* the age-related muscle-shriveling resulting from a sedentary lifestyle
- alter the stereotype of aging as an unalterable process of decline

Len was convinced, and started on my recommended program of thrice-weekly, twenty-minute strength-training sessions. In six weeks he came back to tell me that his fatigue was gone.

"Not only can I begin work early in the morning, my energy doesn't diminish over the course of the day and my evenings are super. And you know what—my body has changed already. I'm still running at the gym, but the addition of weights has made a difference I didn't think was possible. You know, when you first recommended weight training, I thought that was just for guys who are always looking at themselves in the mirror. I was initially afraid I would turn into some muscle-bound bodybuilder."

I told Len that I regularly trained with weights and had not developed the distorted physique he apparently feared. Fifteen years ago I had focused on aerobic exercise for cardiovascular fitness. Several times a week I had run laps in the park or played tennis. At that time, I regarded muscle building as something appropriate only for potential Mr. Universe candidates. But then I hurt my lower back playing tennis, and my focus shifted to resistance training to build up strength. To my great surprise, I discovered that weight training offered benefits that my aerobic workouts could not begin to approach.

Primarily, I found that my stamina increased. I could work longer hours without tiring. Fatigue, always lurking in the shadows of a long, difficult day, did not appear. Working out at a local gym three days a week, I felt stronger, both physically and mentally. Other weight trainers provided inspiration and encouragement, helping me to set new goals and showing me how to attain them safely. As I progressed, I saw clearly the implications weight training could have for my patients who were basically in good physical shape but needed to enhance their endurance.

Len was only one of a number of my patients whose views on weight training changed dramatically, once they started my specially developed weight training program. Jean's experience was a little different.

A regular tennis player who ran in local 5K races and took a weekly yoga class for relaxation and flexibility, Jean was starting to feel fatigue creeping up on her. Her MicroFit Endurance Evaluation showed that her cardiovascular system was functioning extremely well, but that her muscular strength was lacking. While her weight was okay, her percentage of body fat could have been better. And despite her best efforts—and she worked hard at maintaining her workouts—her triceps were flabby, a trait that appeared in all the women in her family. To disguise her upper arms, she had started wearing shirts with larger sleeves; to try to reduce them, she had begun to cut back on her food intake, hoping that would help. It hadn't.

When she pointed out her concerns to me and I suggested endurance training, she was stunned.

"Weight lifters gain weight!" she exclaimed.

I told her that, unlike her regular exercise, endurance training could target her problem areas, tightening, toning, and contouring them. And as for putting on weight, the answer was this: The dial on the scale might go a little higher up—but it would reflect muscle weight, not body fat. And no matter what the scale said, her waistline might actually decrease.

Within two weeks of starting my program, Jean began to see changes. Her energy was back, in full force. And there was an extra plus as well: Her triceps had been firmed, and there was new definition in her upper arms. Striking a balance between her aerobic exercise and resistance training led her to make some interesting observations.

"When I exercise without weight training—for instance, when I run, in-line skate, play tennis, or swim—I feel like I'm fighting my body, which is always trying to get back to a higher weight. I watch what I eat very carefully, and I make sure I'm active to burn up the calories. But the regular twenty-minute strength-training sessions you put me on make me feel as though I've crossed an athletic line. I've never looked, or felt, better. My energy levels have increased, and I never flag during the day. The best thing is that I can eat more—in fact, I've increased my daily intake by an extra four hundred calories!"

Resistance to Resistance Training

Despite the fact that most of my patients are very exercise-savvy, they have as many preconceived—and erroneous—misconceptions about resistance training as anyone else.

Women worry that they will develop bulging muscles

adorned with popping veins if they lift weights regularly. They won't, because women have minuscule levels of testosterone, the male sex hormone responsible for increasing muscle size. Therefore, they cannot build the bulk of a male bodybuilder—unless they take anabolic steroid drugs to artificially induce muscle growth, or train with weights for a minimum of two hours a day, six or seven days a week. Weight training helps women to become stronger, shapelier, and, once their body fat is lowered, more defined.

Frankly, instead of being afraid of acquiring big muscles, both men and women should be more concerned about not having *enough* muscle! Without regular weight training, even the most dedicated aerobic exercisers will gradually lose muscle mass as they age. It is estimated that nonactive men and women will lose one pound of muscle every two years after the age of twenty, or about 5 percent each decade. This is the primary reason why so many people add fat year after year. It's a simple and sobering fact: Less muscle tissue burns fewer calories, and you store the rest as fat.

The Myofibril Connection

Muscle fibers consist of myofibrils, numerous tiny fibers composed of rodlike structures one micrometer in diameter. Myofibrils are made up of strands of protein arranged in units known as sarcomeres. These have sheaths of thin filaments made of actin, a protein, which slides over a thicker fiber made of the protein myosin. It is the constant sliding of the thin over the thicker filaments, triggered by calcium ions that flood into the muscle fiber, that causes a muscle to contract.

From childhood to your twenties, the number of myofibrils in each fiber increases in size, causing muscles to get bigger. However, as you get older, the number of myofibrils slowly begins to drop off, and muscles begin to shrink. Also, muscle fibers lose their sensitivity to calcium ion stimulation, which is critical to growth, adding further to the body's decline.

If you don't take the right steps to correct this process, your muscle will adapt to inactivity. The muscles of a sedentary person begin to shrink. *As much as 40 percent of their mass can be lost in just a few weeks.*

The good news is that our myofibrils can be regenerated by regularly lifting weights at our maximum capacity, defined as the highest amount of weight you can lift eight times in a row for at least twenty minutes, three times a week. Your muscles soon begin to respond. Most of us can attain the maximal increase in muscle-fiber size within six to ten weeks of beginning a regular strength-training program. The need for such a program applies to runners, swimmers, tennis players, and anyone else who is active, as well as to the sedentary.

I tell my patients that working with weights will give them a powerful tool that will help them perform their daily challenges with vigor and concentration. The greater your muscle strength, the less likely you are to become fatigued. And because muscles are the body's furnace, you'll burn more fat, using up to as many as three hundred to four hundred extra calories daily.

When to Begin

Age is not a factor when it comes to endurance training. Dr. William Evans, at the Human Nutrition Research Center on Aging at Tufts University, proved this in his long-term study. He wanted to see whether a modest strength-training program could counteract the muscle weakness and frailty that is all too typical in older people. Working on weight machines three times a week for several months, the seventy-, eighty-, and ninety-year-old participants who took part in the groundbreaking study astonished themselves as well as the scientists observing them. Incredibly, each person:

- doubled muscle strength
- increased daily physical activity, on average, by 35 percent

What this important study so clearly made evident was this:

- While the aging process cannot be stopped, its more pronounced effects can be overcome through muscle strengthening.
- Growing weaker is not a consequence of aging, but rather the result of not using muscles optimally.

The MicroFit Endurance Evaluation

I use a special computerized series of tests made by MicroFit to determine the endurance levels of my patients. This MicroFit Endurance Evaluation is a state-of-the-art appraisal that takes about thirty minutes. It gives a complete profile showing:

- body fat
- body weight
- cardiovascular endurance
- exercise heart rate
- flexibility
- blood pressure
- muscular endurance

The MicroFit system was developed in 1986 by Paul Voda, an exercise physiologist who worked with the Stanford Heart Disease Prevention Program in Palo Alto, California. Simply stated, his MicroFit device is a mini-physiology lab that feeds test results from key physical exams into a computer. The profile results appear on the MicroFit computer screen and are then included in a personalized printout report which compares the patient with other people of the same age and sex.

The MicroFit Endurance Evaluation is extremely accurate; all profile procedures use internationally accepted measurement standards from the American College of Sports Medicine. After starting a patient on my endurance program, I generally schedule a follow-up evaluation to take place within the next three to four months. The second profile shows the progress made as a result of the program.

The MicroFit Endurance Evaluation is currently being used in hundreds of medical facilities around the United States. To find a convenient location near you, call MicroFit at 1-800-822-0405 and ask to speak to Rob Rideout, vice president of sales for MicroFit.

MicroFit Endurance Profile

The following MicroFit profile is of Bonnie Smith, one of my Vitality Medicine patients. At fifty-five, she is extremely encouraged by her results, but also sees specific areas where she can improve her overall endurance. Bonnie is concerned about increasing her muscular strength and feels that her aerobic capacity should also be greater. She is excited by the prospect of periodic retesting to see whether or not she will reach her goals.

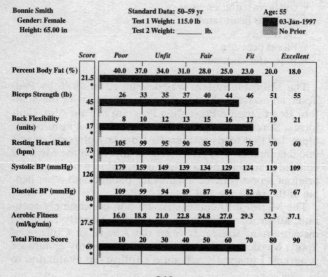

Bonnie Smith
Gender: Female
Height: 65.00 in

Standard Data: 50–59 yr
Test 1 Weight: 115.0 lb
Test 2 Weight: _____ lb.

Age: 55
03-Jan-1997
No Prior

	Score	Poor			Unfit		Fair		Fit		Excellent
Percent Body Fat (%)	21.5	40.0	37.0	34.0	31.0	28.0	25.0	23.0	20.0	18.0
Biceps Strength (lb)	45	26	33	35	37	40	44	46	51	55
Back Flexibility (units)	17	8	10	12	13	15	16	17	19	21
Resting Heart Rate (bpm)	73	105	99	95	90	85	80	75	70	60
Systolic BP (mmHg)	126	179	159	149	139	134	129	124	119	109
Diastolic BP (mmHg)	80	109	99	94	89	87	84	82	79	67
Aerobic Fitness (ml/kg/min)	27.5	16.0	18.8	21.0	22.8	24.8	27.0	29.3	32.3	37.1
Total Fitness Score	69	10	20	30	40	50	60	70	80	90

What the Results Mean

Body fat refers to the percentage of your body weight that is composed of this substance.

Biceps strength is defined as upper body strength measured during an isometric contraction, that is, the maximal force generated against an immovable object. The results may be greater than the maximal amount of weight that can be lifted using other strength equipment. To perform the test, the participant pulls up steadily on a steel bar for five seconds.

Flexibility of the lower back, as well as that of the muscles of the upper back of the legs, is evaluated by performing the sit-and-reach test. The more flexible you are, the greater your ability to engage your muscles and joints through their full range of motion. Optimal flexibility also is critical for good posture. To perform the test, the participant sits on a mat and reaches forward as far as he or she can.

Resting heart rate is the measurement of the organ's regular beating when you are not exercising.

Blood pressure has two measurements, systolic and diastolic, which I will explain shortly. It is evaluated with a standard blood pressure device.

Aerobic endurance defines your level of endurance or stamina, evaluated by gauging your heart rate both at rest and during bicycle exercise. Strong aerobic endurance translates into more calories burned, assisting in both weight loss and maintenance. To perform the test, the participant sits on a stationary bicycle with a heart rate monitor strapped around his or her chest. After a warm-up period, resistance is gradually increased. The heart rate is then monitored and registered at this more strenuous workload.

Total score is a composite of all the test results.

Interpretation of MicroFit Profile Results for Bonnie Smith

Percent Fat: Bonnie's body fat content is 21.5 percent of her body weight. This percent body fat score is in the Fit category. No weight loss is recommended unless desired for aesthetics or athletic performance. To maintain her present percent body fat, Bonnie needs to perform regular aerobic exercise and maintain a diet where the calories from fat are less than 30 percent of total calories consumed.

Muscular Strength: It is important to maintain good muscular strength so you can perform daily activities without fatigue, residual soreness, or risk of injury.

Bonnie's biceps strength score of forty-five pounds is in the Fit category. Performing strength training exercises two days a week will help her to maintain muscular strength while three to four days a week of strength training will improve her overall strength. A complete strength training program should include exercises that involve lifting, pushing, pulling, and leg work.

Flexibility: Maintaining good flexibility is important for good posture, efficient body movement, and reduced risk of muscle and joint injury. Bonnie's back flexibility score of 17 is in the Fit category. To maintain flexibility, she needs to perform stretching exercises three days a week, while stretching four to seven days a week will improve flexibility. Exercises that stretch the muscles and ligaments in the shoulders, back, hip, and legs should be selected. Stretch the target area to a point of discomfort and hold for fifteen to thirty seconds. Repeat each stretch three to five times.

Resting Heart Rate: Resting heart rate is an indicator of health. A high resting heart rate may be a symptom of poor health, while a low resting heart rate confirms normal condition. Bonnie's resting heart rate of 73 beats per minute is in the Fit category. Aerobic exercise can strengthen the heart muscle so it pushes more blood, with each beat resulting in a lower heart rate.

Blood Pressure: Blood pressure is normally reported as systolic pressure over diastolic pressure. The systolic pressure is the higher pressure that occurs when the heart contracts and pushes blood into the arteries. Diastolic pressure is the lower pressure that occurs between contractions when the heart is at rest.

Once again, Bonnie's result falls into the Fit category, with an excellent blood pressure of 126/80. A constant high systolic or diastolic blood pressure increases your risk of heart attack or stroke. Blood pressure below 140/90 is in the normal range. A blood pressure of 160/100 or higher is too high and warrants an immediate visit to a doctor. Blood pressures between normal and high are not cause for alarm, but should be lowered. Actions you can take to lower blood pressure include maintaining ideal body fat, reducing salt intake, and performing regular aerobic exercise.

Aerobic Fitness: Aerobic fitness defines your capacity to sustain long periods of muscular activity such as walking, running, or cycling. Achieving the Fit category is beneficial because daily activities can be performed with little effort and leave a bigger reserve for emergency situations.

Bonnie's aerobic fitness score of 27.5 ml/kg/min is in the Fit category. To maintain and even improve her aerobic fitness, she needs to perform activities such as running, cycling, or swimming three to five days a week for twenty to sixty minutes a day.

Total Fitness Score: The Total Fitness Score is a composite score of all test results, where 98 is the highest score possible and 2 is the lowest. A score between 60 and 80 is recommended for superior stamina and endurance.

Assessing Your Endurance at Home

If you don't want to wait to take a MicroFit Endurance Evaluation, here are three simple home tests that will do an excellent job of helping you to assess your overall stamina. The first assesses the aerobic endurance of your heart and lungs, while the second measures muscular endurance. The third is an evaluation of your flexibility.

1. Aerobic Endurance

The step test is a reliable indicator of your cardiovascular endurance and your general health. You need a stopwatch, comfortable exercise shoes, and a hard surface to step on that is at least eight inches higher than the floor. An actual staircase step will do.

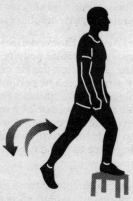

To take the three-minute step test:

Stand in front of the step.

Step up with your right leg, following with your left.

Step down on your right leg, following with your left. Your aim is to complete two up-and-down cycles in five seconds.

Step up and down for three minutes without stopping.

Sit down and rest for thirty seconds.

Take your pulse for thirty seconds. Place your index and middle fingers just below the base of the thumb and just above the tendons on the opposite arm. Move your fingertips around until you locate a strong, steady pulse.

Compare your results to the chart on the next page.

Note: If you are too exhausted at any time during the test, do not continue it. Score yourself in the poor category, which means that your aerobic endurance is at its lowest level. Your aim is to complete three thirty-minute aerobic endurance sessions a week (for instance, walking, running, swimming, cycling, in-line skating) with a day of rest in between each one to allow your muscles needed recovery time.

After a month, repeat the step test. You should now be able to complete it, proving that your aerobic endurance has been increased substantially.

THREE-MINUTE STEP TEST RESULTS: FOR MEN

Age	30–39	40–49	50+
	Number of Beats for 30 Seconds		
Excellent	35–38	37–39	37–40
Good	39–41	40–42	41–43
Average	42–43	43–44	44–45
Fair	44–47	45–49	46–49
Poor	48–59	50–60	50–62

THREE-MINUTE STEP TEST RESULTS: FOR WOMEN

Age	30–39	40–49	50+
	Number of Beats for 30 Seconds		
Excellent	39–42	41–43	41–44
Good	43–45	44–45	45–47
Average	46–47	46–47	48–49
Fair	48–53	48–54	50–55
Poor	54–66	55–67	56–66

2. Muscular Endurance

You can easily measure the overall muscular endurance of your upper, middle, and lower body with the following three basic tests. Check your scores against the chart below to determine your current muscular strength. These scores are for men in their thirties; women's scores will be approximately 20 percent less than for men. On average, scores will decrease approximately 15 percent each decade.

ENDURANCE TEST RESULTS

Wall Sit	Abdominal Hold	Push-ups
High: 77 seconds	High: 21 seconds	High: 21
Average: 51 seconds	Average: 13 seconds	Average: 13
Low: under 26 seconds	Low: under 4 seconds	Low: less than 4

a. The Wall Sit

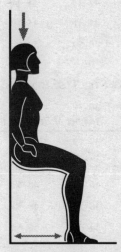

This test measures the strength of your thigh muscles. To perform it, stand and lean your back against a wall. Your feet, flat on the floor and shoulder-width apart, should be approximately six inches from the wall. Gently slide down the wall until your upper thighs are approximately at a forty-five-degree angle to the floor and you are in a sitting position. Hold this position for as long as you can.

b. *The Abdominal Hold*

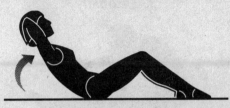

This exercise determines the strength of your abdominal muscles. Strong muscles in this area are important for good posture and for preventing lower back problems. Lie on your back on the floor with your knees bent at a forty-five degree angle. Your feet should be flat on the floor. Keeping your fingers interlaced behind your head, raise your shoulders off the floor until they form a forty-five-degree angle with the floor. Hold this position for as long as you can.

c. *The Push-up*

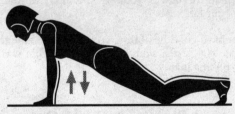

This is a test of upper-body strength. Men should perform as many complete regular push-ups as they are able. Women should do this modified version:

Lie facedown on the floor, your legs together. Keep your hands at the sides of your chest, palms flat on the floor. Straighten your arms out, keep your back flat, and, using your knees as the pivot point, push your upper legs and chest off the floor. Lower yourself back down to the floor, touching the floor only with your chin. Your chest, abdomen, and thighs should not touch the floor. This counts as one repetition. Repeat as many as you can while maintaining the proper push-up form.

3. *Flexibility*

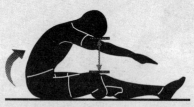

This exercise will test the flexibility of your hamstring muscles (located on the backs of your thighs) and is a good indicator of overall muscle flexibility. To perform it:

Sit on the floor. Extend your left leg straight out in front of you.

Bend your right leg so that the sole of your right foot touches the inside of your left knee.

Gently lean forward at your waist and try to touch your head to your left knee.

If you have good flexibility, you should be able to touch your knee if you're a woman, and come within two inches of it if you're a man.

A Baseline to Build On

Once you know your baseline endurance levels, you have a basic foundation on which to build. Retake the tests regularly every three months and compare the outcomes with the original results so you can chart your progress. Remember that a high score in one element of endurance doesn't balance out a poor score in another. Your overall goal is to have maximum endurance and score well in each test. One of the best ways I have found to help increase overall endurance is with my 7/20 program.

The 7/20 Endurance Program
(Seven Activities in Twenty Minutes)

Time is a valuable commodity, and making the best use of it is vitally important to my patients and myself. Building endurance should fit into the time constraints of active people, and the 7/20 Endurance Program does just that. Michael Margulies, the director of the Med Fitness facility in New York, works with many of my patients and has found the 7/20 program to be an extremely effective twenty-minute fatigue-busting, endurance-boosting workout. The program can be done at home three times a week. Both men and women can obtain excellent results using it. One of the best things about the program is that it maximizes endurance benefits while it minimizes equipment required. You will need dumbbells (for as little as $100), an exercise bench (about $100–$200), and a pull-up bar ($10–$25). If you don't want to invest in the exercise bench, you can substitute a shoulder-width table or, if it has a level, solid seat, a chair.

The regimen has three specific aims. It will:

1. Increase overall endurance.
2. Fortify the muscles of the upper body, particularly the biceps and triceps.
3. Strengthen the muscles in the lower body, especially the thighs.

The seven weight training activities will give you the stamina you need to carry you through your busy life. The program includes time for a warm-up period to loosen the muscles as well as a cool-down period to keep the muscles from tightening up postworkout, which helps to prevent injury.

This is a basic beginner's program. If you are a longtime weight trainer who works out regularly, this information may seem elementary. I suggest that you read it anyway. There may be information that is new to you.

One Set for Strength and Power

For decades, three sets of ten repetitions each was the gospel for each weight-training activity. Now, research has proven this maxim obsolete. *What this means is that a great endurance workout is now possible by doing a lot less. You will accomplish more, and finish up a lot earlier, than ever before.*

According to results from a study at the University of Florida, performing one set of each exercise during a weight-training session means achieving the same strength gains equal to three sets. According to Michael Pollock, Ph.D., the director of the university's Center for Exercise Science, *there is no need to do more than one set in order to attain substantial gains or to maintain current levels of strength.*

In his research, Dr. Pollock put forty adults through a fourteen-week strength-training program. Twenty-two of the subjects performed a single set (eight to twelve repetitions) of a specific exercise three times a week. The other eighteen did three sets of the same exercise. He then compared the outcome of both groups with a control group of ten who didn't exercise at all.

Not surprisingly, the control group exhibited no gains in strength. But to Dr. Pollock's surprise, both weight-lifting groups made similar gains in power and muscle thickness.

The Four Keys to Endurance Training

Consistent endurance training can impose wonderful health benefits. But in order to ensure that progress is made safely and methodically, you need to follow the four basic training keys.

1. Pick a weight you can lift at least ten consecutive times but no more than twelve times.

A repetition (or "rep") is one complete cycle of lifting and lowering a weight. The last repetition should be difficult to do.

If you are just starting out, take it easy. If you find that you are struggling with the weight on repetitions five through ten, then you are using too much weight; reduce it by five pounds. If you are using less than five-pound weights to start and don't have a smaller weight, cut back your repetitions to five until you get stronger. Gradually work up to ten or twelve reps without straining.

When you can do twelve repetitions with a particular weight for two sessions in a row, increase the weight just enough so that you can handle ten reps at the new weight.

Remember: You will make big gains by making small, gradual increases in weight.

2. Lift weights in a slow, controlled fashion.

Be sure to learn the correct movement for each exercise. Inhale at the beginning of the lift, slowly exhaling until you finish the repetition. Each rep should take at least five seconds to complete.

3. Perform one set of each exercise.

A "set" is a predetermined number of repetitions of an exercise. I have found that the best results for building endurance comes from performing one set of ten repetitions for each exercise. Using this as the foundation of the program, it should take you approximately twenty minutes to perform the seven exercises.

4. Perform your resistance training three times a week, with one rest day in between.

This will allow for adequate muscle recovery and growth. When you exercise vigorously, your muscle fibers are injured slightly, causing them to feel sore eight to twenty-four hours after the workout. When muscle fibers are damaged, white blood cells release a protein called interleukin-2, which prompts the hurt cells to release prostaglandins, causing the pain. However, they also begin the healing process. If you train the same muscles day after day without a rest, this muscle breakdown/growth process is interrupted and it will be difficult to accomplish optimal gains.

PowerBlock: The Essential Equipment

For the 7/20 endurance-building regimen, I recommend a specific set of dumbbells. I have found the PowerBlock to be the perfect home strength-training unit because of its ease of operation. Just slide the selector pin into the block and lift out a weight, from five to forty-five pounds. Offering variety, efficiency, and comfort, the PowerBlock barely takes up any space. My two New York City phone books are actually bulkier.

The ingenious PowerBlock weight system (Intellbell, Inc., 2020 Austin Road, Owatonna, Minnesota 55060; tel. 1-800-446-5215) is the equivalent of sixteen pairs of dumbbells conveniently compressed into two hand-held adjustable weight stacks.

The 7/20 Endurance-Building Workout

Perform one set of eight to twelve repetitions for each exercise. Even though the workout takes less than half an hour, don't rush through it. The program was designed to provide superior results when done at a steady pace for twenty minutes.

Remember: If you suddenly feel tired at any time during the 7/20 program, stop and take a rest before continuing. Extreme weariness means that you're exercising too hard. Your body needs to slow down.

The Warm-up

Begin the program with a two-to-three-minute warm-up. This will slowly raise your heart and breathing rate, increase blood flow to the muscles, open the lungs, and prepare your muscles for the demands of the workout. Good choices include jogging in place at an easy pace, skipping rope, or a brisk walk. After warming up, lightly stretch your arms and legs, as well as any muscles that may be stiff. Warmed-up muscles accumulate less lactic acid, which means less fatigue.

After your warm-up, follow the sequence as follows:

1. Dumbbell Bench Press

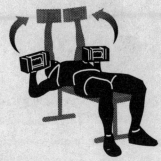

(Works the shoulder and chest muscles)

Lie on your back on an exercise bench with your feet flat on the floor.

Hold a dumbbell in each hand, palms facing forward, elbows bent so that the weights are at your side.

Slowly raise both dumbbells straight up until your arms are fully extended directly above your chest.

Slowly lower the weights.

Repeat.

2. *Lunge with Dumbbells*

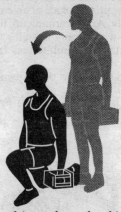

(Works the quadriceps, buttocks, thighs, and lower back muscles)

Stand with your back straight and your feet about eight inches apart.

Hold a dumbbell in each hand with your palms facing your sides.

Take a large step forward with your left foot.

Lower your right knee until it almost touches the floor. Make sure that the toes of your right foot do not leave the floor.

Return slowly to the starting position.

Repeat the lunge with your right leg.

3. *Dumbbell Kick Backs*

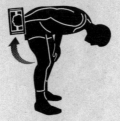

(Works the triceps)

Hold a dumbbell in your right hand.

Bend over at your waist until your chest is parallel to the floor.

Place your left hand on your left knee.

Press your entire right arm to your side, keeping it vertical.

Press the dumbbell back until your entire arm is horizontal.

Lower the weight to the starting position and repeat.

When finished with the right arm, repeat with your left.

4. Dumbbell Military Press

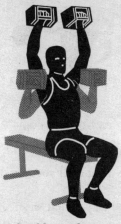

(Works shoulder and arm muscles)

Hold a pair of dumbbells in your hands.

Sit on an exercise bench or chair with your feet flat on the floor.

Let your arms hang freely, palms facing inward toward your thighs.

Raise the dumbbells slowly to the starting position at shoulder height. Face your palms forward.

Push the weights straight up almost to full arm extension.

Pause momentarily and then slowly lower the weight to the starting position.

Repeat.

5. Overhead Extension

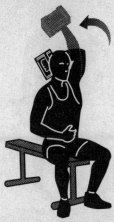

(Works triceps and abdominal muscles)

Sit on a chair or an exercise bench with your back straight, feet flat on the floor.

Hold a dumbbell in your left hand.

Raise the dumbbell to the starting position above your head, palm facing forward.

Slowly lower the weight behind your head by bending your elbow. Stop when your forearm touches your biceps.

Raise the dumbbell until your arm is fully extended overhead.

Repeat and then perform the exercise with your other arm.

6. Biceps Curl

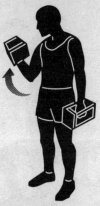

(Works biceps)

Stand with your back straight, feet shoulder-width apart, dumbbells held in each hand, palms facing inward at your sides.

Turn your palms to face forward, bend at your elbows, and raise the weights up until they touch your shoulders.

Slowly lower them to the starting position.

Repeat.

7. Pull-Up

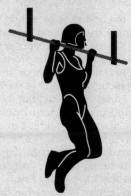

(Works the arm, shoulder, and abdominal muscles)

Grasp a pull-up bar with palms facing forward, hands wider than shoulder width.

Pull yourself up until your chin reaches the bar.

Lower and repeat five times. (This may require the assistance of a training partner to give a helpful boost in order to complete the pull-ups.)

The Cool-Down

Intense activity can cause your heart and lungs to pump at twice their normal pace. If you stop your workout suddenly, blood may pool in the dilated vessels of your legs. This can lead to a quick bout of dizziness. You can avoid this by spending two to five minutes cooling down. Good choices include performing some of the 7/20 exercises with the lightest weight, taking a five-minute walk, or executing a few of your favorite gentle stretches.

The Circadian Advantage

For most people, the best time to weight train, that is, the time when your body will respond most effectively, is between 5:00 and 6:00 P.M. One exception would be people with diabetes and others who suffer from low blood sugar, in which case the best time is one hour after meals.

For reasons of practicality, many of us must schedule our workout sessions around work and family obligations. I do this myself. While I much prefer to weight train around 5:00 P.M., it's not always possible. I've discovered that, while my later evening sessions are certainly beneficial, they are not so satisfying as their earlier counterpart. For instance, I find that during the later program I feel fatigued, and I can't push as much weight as I usually do. Also, I tire more easily. When I return to the earlier time I have a superior session.

It's not so hard to schedule this "time-out" as you may think. Hilary, a very busy psychotherapist, locks her office door three times a week at 5:00 P.M. Between patients, she performs her twenty-minute weight-training session. Not only does it energize her for the rest of her workday; she doesn't have to leave the premises to work out because she keeps a set of dumbbells in her office.

I do the same thing myself, as a backup position to those times when it's just not possible to get to the gym at the preferred hour. Other times, I'll just lace on my boxing gloves and hit the heavy bag I have hanging from my bedroom ceiling for fifteen minutes or so. But, of course, what is most important is to have a set time for your regime that guarantees you will work out regularly. If you can do it in the afternoon or early evening, so much the better.

Why Time of Day Matters

The reason for the disparity between good and not-as-effective training is related to our daily rhythmic activity cycle, known as circadian rhythm.

All of us have our own circadian rhythms, which have a

direct effect on certain body cycles, including temperature and heart rate, blood pressure, and hormone release. The usual body temperature starts at a low 97°F. range before 7:00 A.M., and then rises rapidly to 98.6°F. It holds steady until about 6:00 P.M., and then it starts to drop again. If you do your weight training after your temperature begins its decline, your efforts will be under par.

Circadian researchers have determined that the hours between 3:00 and 6:00 P.M. are the best for body training. Most top athletes have an awareness of their circadian rhythms, and train accordingly. In a study of Olympic and Division 1 NCAA athletes, Dr. Roger Smith of the Sleep Disorders Clinic and Research Center at Stanford University School of Medicine recently found that:

- Only slightly more than 20 percent of his subjects peaked athletically between 9:00 a.m. and noon.
- Sixty percent of the subjects were at their athletic peak between 3:00 P.M. and 6:00 P.M.
- Fewer than 20 percent trained between 6:00 and 9:00 P.M.
- No one had satisfactory workouts before 9:00 a.m. or after 9:00 p.m.

My advice for maximizing peak performance training is to use your natural circadian advantage whenever you can. If it's at all possible in your busy day, plan your endurance training for the late afternoon. At that time, your strength, body, and flexibility are all at their peaks.

The Ergogenic Program

Ergogenic, from the Greek *ergon,* which means work, is the term I use to describe any method for enhancing endurance. I apply it to improving energy utilization, delaying fatigue, and building muscle.

In addition to my specific stamina-building physical program, I also recommend the use of particular ergogenic enhancers. These protein builders, HMB, creatine, branched-chain amino acids, and ciwujia can help to fortify muscles, hold off fatigue, reduce body fat, and improve the overall ability to get through any day, no matter how demanding it is.

The sequence of endurance training works like this. Lifting weights will yield results based on the energy expended to do them. Once you perform your program long enough, you'll likely want the extra edge, which will boost results even more. This is where HMB, creatine, branched-chain amino acids, and ciwujia, the ergogenic enhancers, come in.

While this quartet is relatively new in this country, ergogenic aids are not. Specific substances utilized to boost and maximize performance have been used for thousands of years. In fact, the early consumption of animal flesh by man may have actually started as an attempt to possess the power of a given animal.

Over the centuries, elixirs, potions, teas, and tonics of all varieties have been used in an effort to build strength. They continue to be used in this manner in increasing numbers today by an ever-broadening segment of the population. Interestingly, even when mortality rates dropped and lifespans increased, the use of ergogenic enhancers did not disappear from use. Today, they continue to be sought by those seeking an additional "edge." The most effective substances in use now were studied in both athletes and soldiers, two groups of people who continually push themselves to achieve ever greater performance levels.

Now others who aspire to battle fatigue and build bigger, stronger muscles can turn to safe, natural mixtures of nutritional supplements to help them achieve their goals. When used in conjunction with consistent weight training, these ergogenic enhancers offer a reliable method of achieving maximum strength and muscle development. Each substance:

- is a naturally-occurring amino acid or herbal extract
- has been tested extensively and found to be safe and side-effect free
- has produced significant, documented results which I observe on a daily basis

This has happened over and over again with patients who had not worked with weights regularly or with particular skill.

"I went from bench-pressing barely ninety-five pounds to being able to press close to 150 pounds in less than two months, and my percentage of body fat has dropped by 5 percent," a forty-three-year-old man reported. He was taking HMB.

"I've been lifting weights for almost ten years but I shied away from any supplements; I thought they would do strange things to my body," a forty-six-year-old woman told me. "But now I want to reach the personal best I had eight years ago." She began taking creatine, and within six weeks she had achieved her goal. Two weeks after that, she hit a new personal record.

"I've noticed a one-inch increase in the circumference of my biceps and my thighs after one month of taking branched-chain amino acids," a thirty-seven-year-old man stated.

"I've never experienced such intense training sessions since I've started using branched-chain amino acids," a forty-nine-year-old woman told me. "Instead of feeling stiff and a bit sore after training, I now feel pumped. I'm relaxed, as if I had just had a swim, and hadn't lifted weights at all."

"My running workouts—and I've been doing them for years—have never felt so effortless," said a fifty-one-year-old man after he started taking ciwujia, an herb from China.

HMB: What It Is

Muscle-building supplements have been available for centuries, but most of them were ineffective. Those that worked caused serious side effects. But HMB (which stands for beta-hydroxy-methylbutyrate) falls into neither category. A substance required to repair muscle tissue, HMB is produced normally in small amounts by the body through protein metabolism. However, in 1995, a patented synthetic form of HMB became available. It not only protects the muscles during endurance activities; it aids in rapid muscle growth as well.

Double-blind studies with athletes who supplemented their daily diets with 3g of HMB, the amount of protein contained in 500 g of red meat, showed that the athletes gained 63 percent more size and muscle strength than exercisers who received a placebo. Additionally, test subjects in this tightly controlled study lost more than twice as much fat as those who did not use HMB but who followed the same exercise and nutrition program.

According to Dr. Naji Abumrad, the chief of surgery at North Shore Health System in Long Island, who helped direct the double-blind research trials with human subjects, HMB is not a steroid. Nor is it classified as a drug. Rather, it is a nutritional substance made from proteins containing the amino acid leucine.

Leucine is found in all dietary protein and is an essential building block of protein in all tissue. HMB supplements deliver a pure leucine metabolite. This differs from protein supplements (drinks, shakes, powders, and pills) that provide many amino acids that must then compete on a cellular level, often negating the effectiveness of a single amino acid. The truly unique characteristic of leucine is that it helps regulate protein synthesis and breakdown.

Why not just take extra leucine? Won't it have the same effects as HMB? The answer to both questions is no. In order for the body to make 3 g of HMB, an effective muscle-protective dose, you would have to take at least 60 g of leucine daily. Besides being expensive and impractical, it would trigger immediate and severe stomach distress.

"HMB is produced in small quantities in the body. Under stressful situations, a human can't synthesize enough HMB in the body to meet the needs of the muscles," says Dr. Abumrad. "However, by supplementing your diet with HMB you can help to stimulate muscle growth safely and effectively."

In the extensive animal and human studies Dr. Abumrad has conducted with HMB, there have been no signs of HMB toxicity at any level.

How Muscles Get Bigger

Made up primarily of protein (amino acids) and water, muscles grow in a process that consists of synthesizing and breaking down protein. The actual growth of muscle depends, in large part, on how much protein is made and how much is broken down. If bigger and stronger muscles are your goal, you must alter your body's existing protein cycle. There are two ways to do this: Speed up the rate of protein synthesis or slow down the rate of protein breakdown.

Anabolic steroids, known muscle builders, work by altering the body's protein balance. They protect muscle cells from cortisol, the hormone that breaks down protein. Legal issues and sporting ethics aside, the problem with anabolic steroids is a medical one: They can have serious side effects.

The HMB Effect

HMB was discovered in 1988 by Dr. Steven Nissen, a veterinarian and professor of animal science at Iowa State University. In fact, he holds the patent on HMB manufacture. His research team found that supplements of HMB appeared to burn fat during exercise. Human studies showed that HMB also increased the body's natural potential to build muscle during exercise. It did this by minimizing the muscle tissue breakdown that occurs naturally after a weight-training workout.

For anyone wanting to build muscle size and strength responsibly, HMB supplementation is the safe choice. Using it can benefit virtually any adult who weight trains on a regular basis. It is especially helpful for those people who become frustrated by their lack of progress and are thinking of abandoning their training.

The Supporting Research

Extensively researched and tested on animals by Dr. Nissen, HMB has been shown to maximize growth and prevent muscle loss due to the negative effects of stress.

In stressful situations, the adrenal gland is stimulated to

release the hormone cortisol which, among other things, provokes muscle protein loss and suppression of the immune system. However, when Dr. Nissen administered HMB to his animals, it safely counteracted these harmful outcomes, leading to significant increases in growth as well as improved overall health.

When this conclusive animal testing was finished, Dr. Nissen began to study the effects of HMB on humans. Forty-one male volunteers between the ages of nineteen and twenty-nine were recruited. Each one followed the same weight-training program, which included the use of both free weights and machines, and alternated between upper and lower body exercises. The test subjects worked out three times a week, with at least one day of rest between sessions. Their nutrition intake was carefully monitored. On average, every day the men consumed approximately 2,400 calories, and between 117 and 175 g of protein.

After the first week, in which all the test subjects exercised together, fifteen of them were given 3 g of HMB every day, thirteen received 1.5 g of HMB daily, and the control group of thirteen had no HMB. The researchers monitored the volunteers extensively during this period, and it became immediately obvious that the use of HMB was producing dramatic results. After just one week, the muscle protein breakdown in the group receiving 3 g of HMB had decreased by 44 percent. As the study proceeded, muscle protein breakdown continued to be considerably lower than that of the other two groups.

By the time the study was over, the group using 3 g of HMB daily had gained nearly three solid pounds of lean mass, 55 percent more lean mass than the group of nonusers. Additionally, while losing 7.3 percent of body fat (compared to 2.2 percent for the placebo group), they experienced gains in strength that were 295 percent greater than the test subjects who followed the same workout program but did not use HMB at all. And while the results of the group using 1.5 g of HMB were impressive, they paled in comparison to those of the subjects who took 3 g a day of the ergogenic enhancer.

The HMB Facts

I recommend a minimum of 3 g a day of HMB for both men and women, to be taken 1g at a time, morning, noon, and night, with meals.

Remember: Although HMB can help to produce incredible gains in muscle mass, taking it without exercising negates its purpose. To reap its benefits, you need to give your muscles the workout they require.

My patients have asked me a number of questions about ergogenic enhancers. Here are their queries, with answers, about HMB.

1. How does HMB work?

As is the case with so many substances that impart positive benefits on the human body, no one is absolutely sure. One scientific theory posits that HMB helps proteolysis, the natural process of breaking down muscle cells that occurs after strenuous activity. It appears that HMB supplementation may help the body get a head start on its recovery process. This may be very beneficial, especially for those people who really push themselves in their weight-lifting program.

2. Who might benefit from HMB supplementation?

HMB supplementation can work for all adults who are seriously interested in putting on solid muscle and reducing their body fat levels. This recommendation works exceptionally well for those who weight train, and it can be utilized as well by people who combine weight lifting with their overall running, bicycling, and swimming program.

3. Does HMB work as well for women as it does for men?

A study is currently under way at Iowa State University to determine if HMB has the same positive effect in aiding women as it does men. The speculation is that women should see results similar to those men achieve.

4. How long does it take to see effects from HMB?

Studies show that measurable increases in strength and muscle can begin in as little as one week, and three to four weeks will produce dramatic results. You will also notice that your personal fatigue barriers will be extended. For instance, if you normally tire after twenty minutes of training, you will find that taking HMB will lengthen the period of time before you become fatigued.

5. Who should not take HMB?

Pregnant or lactating women are advised against taking HMB because safety studies have not yet been done for this segment of the population. Also, individuals with any known medical problems should consult with their physicians prior to using HMB.

6. Are there any other nutritional supplements that produce effects similar to HMB?

There are many other substances that appear to reduce protein breakdown in the body and may also exert a positive impact on muscle function. These include the branched-chain amino acid leucine, which produces HMB during metabolism, and glutamine. Scientific studies seem to indicate that these amino acids need to be consumed in such high quantities that it makes their use inconvenient and impractical. Thirty g or more of leucine or glutamine may be required, versus 3 g of HMB.

7. Can anabolic steroids or human growth hormone give better and quicker results?

Anabolic steroids, first introduced by track-and-field athletes in the 1960s and used worldwide as an ergogenic training aid and in performance training, are powerful substances. However, they have fallen into disfavor. Not only were these testosterone-based drugs considered unethical; they also caused severe acne, hair loss, vomiting, nausea, permanently enlarged breasts, and diminished libido.

Human growth hormone (hGH), once only available in limited quantities (it was made from the pituitary glands of monkeys), received much wider use when a company named Genentech introduced a synthetic version. The hormone transports amino acids between the cells, helping synthesize protein, thereby strengthening and building muscle. While many athletes took hGH and found they could train longer and develop bigger muscles, they observed unpleasant side effects from long-term use. Carpal tunnel syndrome, diabetes, gynecomastia (breast development in men), and acromegaly (the elongation of bones in the face, arms, and legs) have made hGH a highly undesirable, if not dangerous, ergogenic enhancer.

8. *Where can I purchase HMB?*
HMB is currently available at all GNC health food stores nationwide.

Creatine: What It Is

Like HMB, creatine is available in food and is a component of muscle tissue. A protein found primarily in raw meat and fish, its levels unfortunately plummet once the food source has been cooked.

Produced by our livers (about 2 g per day) from the amino acids arginine and glycine, creatine (pronounced cree-AH-ten) is then transported by the blood and stored in skeletal muscle, the heart, and other body cells. In the muscles, creatine is synthesized into a compound called creatine phosphate.

It is creatine phosphate that helps the body to perform intense exercise, such as lifting weights or sprinting on a bicycle or treadmill. While it does not alter muscle size and structure, creatine improves the ability to maintain maximal performance by fueling the muscles. The high-energy phosphates stored in creatine phosphate help to convert supplies of ADP, or adenosine diphosphate, into ATP, or adenosine triphosphate, the main fuel that allows muscles to contract.

In theory, when the muscles are supersaturated with creatine, there will be more energy available from creatine phosphate for short-duration peak activities. Also, with more creatine phosphate present in the muscles, lactic acid, the muscle by-product that causes fatigue, may be buffered, and the eventual onset of tiredness delayed. With the increase of creatine, you are able to train more intensely, thereby boosting your short-term muscle power and long-term muscle growth.

The Supporting Research

Dr. Bjorn Ekblom, a professor of physiology at the Karolinska Institute in Stockholm, along with several other Swedish scientists, conducted tests to investigate whether creatine supplementation could delay the onset of fatigue during repeated bouts of short-burst, high-intensity exercise.

In one study, eight Swedish physical education students were given creatine supplements for five days, while another group of eight received placebos. Five days later, the subjects performed high-intensity sprints on bicycle ergometers (130 pedal revolutions per minute) for ten seconds, interspersed with thirty seconds of rest. The next day the test was repeated, but this time the pedal revolutions were upped to 140 rpm to induce fatigue more rapidly.

Test results showed conclusively that, while the exercise output of the placebo group decreased, the creatine group was able to sustain a higher pedal frequency over the final few moments of each bout. In both tests, creatine supplementation resulted in lower blood lactate accumulation.

Interestingly, creatine has shown no positive effect during prolonged continuous exercise—and it may actually decrease performance. In Dr. Ekblom's study of eighteen Swedish runners conducted with physiologists Karin Soderlund and Paul Balsom—nine were given creatine for six days and nine received a placebo—ran a rolling six-mile cross-country course prior to and after supplementation. The placebo group maintained or improved their times, while the creatine group, which gained an average of one pound in weight, decreased their running pace. Researchers believe that the added body weight due to water retention caused by the creatine may have been responsible for the slower running time.

Since creatine is a legitimate food supplement that happens to provide large quantities of fuel to the muscles, and because excess creatine is excreted in the urine, the use of this ergogenic enhancer at the recommended dosage does not appear to pose any medical risks.

The use of creatine supplements is still in its early stages, but it is important to know that it has not been banned by either the U.S. or the international Olympic committees. As research continues and more athletes experiment and achieve success with creatine, we may find that it has even greater potential for added strength.

Creatine and the Heart

Creatine supplementation is also being observed with heart patients, especially those with ischemia, or reduced blood flow to the heart. As we age, we naturally produce less creatine, so scientists in England are currently investigating whether supplements, combined with exercise, can help reinforce the heart muscle as well as help improve its overall function.

The Creatine Facts

Initial research with creatine found that the best way to take the supplement involved a special two-part loading phase. Twenty g of creatine were taken daily for six days, and then were followed by a daily maintenance phase of 2 g per day. However, recent research in Sweden investigated this practice and found that it produced equivalent results to those produced when taking a reduced dosage right from the start. Since the exercise scientists found that both supplementation schemes produced similar increases of creatine in the body, the loading phase is now considered unnecessary.

The recommended dose of creatine for both men and women is 3 g a day.

Dissolve 3 g of creatine (about one to two teaspoons) in 8 oz. of fruit juice. The natural sugars in the juice will help create a surge in insulin that will maximize the intake of creatine.

For the most beneficial effect, have the drink before breakfast or right after your training.

Here are the most frequently asked questions about creatine.

1. How do creatine supplements help muscles to grow?
Creatine helps to heighten the intensity of your training program by recycling ATP. By building the body's supply of creatine, you are helping to augment the rate at which your body can supply ATP, the muscle fuel. This supercompensation allows you to work harder, subsequently adding more muscle. Creatine also buffers the development of lactic acid, the main contributor to muscle fatigue.

2. Does creatine work like an anabolic steroid?
No. Creatine is not an anabolic agent; it doesn't directly promote muscle growth.

3. How do I know creatine is working for me?
After the first week of using supplements your muscles should become larger and you should be able to lift heavier weights.

4. Who should not take creatine?
Creatine can be used safely by all adults.

5. Where can I purchase creatine?
Most health food stores nationwide now carry creatine.

Branched-Chain Amino Acids:
What They Are

I was first introduced to branched-chain amino acids by Dr. Francesco Dioguardi, a practicing internist and professor of internal medicine and gastroenterology at the University of Milan. His breakthrough study with athletes on the use of his patented formulation of branched-chain amino acids (BCAAs), which carries the brand name The Big One, had brought him to New York. His formula not only fought off fatigue safely and effectively; it quickly added muscle to the body of anyone who exercised.

BCAAs, along with seventeen other amino acids, are the building blocks that form all of the protein in our bodies. However, the three amino acids—leucine, isoleucine, and valine—in The Big One are site-specific: They go directly to muscle. (Most amino acids need to be processed in the liver first.) Taking the supplement before training helps to double the free fatty acid concentration in the blood in under twenty minutes. This allows the body to shift immediately to the utilization of fats, thereby sparing the glycogen, or sugar, in the muscle for more exercise.

The Supporting Research

Scientists have found that BCAAs are critical for muscle growth and optimal performance enhancement. Leucine, isoleucine, and valine make up 35 percent of the muscle's protein; they are the major components in all muscle building. During regular endurance programs, the trio is broken down and burned for energy. If this happens often enough, muscle protein begins to dwindle, and performance starts to drop. This is why those who take BCAAs do so before and after their training sessions. BCAAs are also used by the muscles to help lower ammonia and lactic acid production, which builds up during training and can lead to post-training stiffness and soreness.

The BCAA Studies

Several studies with athletes reveal that supplemental BCAAs can boost workout and competition performance. For example, after using 24 g daily of The Big One for fifteen days in his study with trained athletes, Dr. Dioguardi noted an increase in biceps circumference of a centimeter or more in the group that took them, when compared to the control group that was not given the BCAAs.

In an Australian university study that measured the effects of BCAAs on endurance, twelve bicyclists were given 12 g of BCAAs every day before pedaling. A control group was given a placebo. The cyclists then rode their bicycles at top speed for two continuous hours. The test was repeated over a period of six days, with blood samples taken regularly to measure enzyme levels for muscle tissue damage. The final results were impressive: Those cyclists who were given the BCAAs performed better and had much less muscle damage than the control group.

BCAAs: The Tryptophan Connection

Tryptophan, along with the vitamins B_6 and B_{12}, helps the brain to manufacture the neurotransmitter serotonin. This brain chemical is responsible for regulating many of our key body functions, from sleep patterns and body temperature to eating habits and mood. It also has an effect on our tolerance for pain. How much tryptophan is in the blood and brain is what ultimately determines the status of your serotonin availability, and, therefore, how fatigued you become when you build endurance.

When you weight train, your BCAAs are slowly used by your muscles. This, in turn, causes the natural levels of tryptophan to begin to rise, increasing serotonin levels in the process. Fatigue is the outcome—and training soon comes to a halt.

Therefore, the key to longer, more effective sessions is to prevent tryptophan from getting into the brain. This can be done by using supplemental BCAAs. The amino acids "flood" the bloodstream, competing with tryptophan for entry through the blood-brain barrier. Tryptophan is overwhelmed and the manufacture of serotonin is decreased. And less serotonin production means increased endurance.

The BCAA Facts

The full range of benefits offered by The Big One, the BCAA supplement developed by Dr. Dioguardi, is currently being investigated in a double-blind study at the Center for Sports Research at Penn State University.

My recommendation for both men and women for improving muscle growth and recovery is to take 20 to 30 g of BCAAs daily, in two equal doses. Take one dose 45 to 120 minutes before endurance training and the second dose within thirty minutes of ending your workout. Note: If you weigh 150 pounds or less, take 10 to 15 g on the same schedule.

For maximum muscle-loading effectiveness, abstain from any drink or food containing sugar two hours before taking the BCAAs and do not take any sugar-containing drink or foods during the workout.

Here are the most asked questions about BCAAs.

1. Should the BCCAs be taken with food?

To derive as much value from them as possible, it is best to take BCAAs on any empty stomach. This way, they won't have to compete with any other proteins for absorption. Also, BCAAs require no digestion.

2. How long will it take before I see a difference in my body?

To begin seeing noticeable results, you must continue with your regular strength training sessions, taking the BCAAs for a minimum of two weeks before and after training. Strength and power gains will be achieved and maintained the longer you continue to use the BCAAs.

3. How will taking BCAAs affect my fatigue?

Using BCAAs allows you to exercise more intensely and longer than ever before, delaying or even preventing noticeable levels of fatigue. Interestingly, many people have reported that their concentration levels increase dramatically with BCAAs. According to Dr. Dioguardi, this is likely due to some unique and positive effect of the BCAAs on various brain receptors.

4. Who should not take BCAAs?

BCAAs can be used safely by all adults. However, those people with liver or kidney disease should consult with their physician first.

5. Where can I purchase BCAAs?

Currently available throughout Italy, The Big One can be ordered directly by contacting Professional Dietetics, Via Menotti 1/A, Milano 20122, Italy (tel. 011-39-2-744-020), or through the Internet at <http://www.docalchemist@

webcity.it>. Also, many health food stores in this country now sell very good BCAA mixtures.

Ciwujia: What It Is

A Chinese root marketed in this country under the name of Endurox, ciwujia (pronounced sue-WAH-jah) is a natural dietary supplement that can increase fat metabolism and improve training performance when taken as part of a normal workout regimen. A nonaddictive ergogenic enhancer, ciwujia has been used for 1,700 years in traditional Chinese medicine to treat fatigue.

Robert Portman, a New Jersey biochemist and founder of PacificHealth Laboratories, became intrigued by the fact that Chinese mountain climbers regularly used this root to improve their stamina at high altitudes. Working closely with Dr. Colin Campbell, a professor of nutritional biochemistry at Cornell University and the director of the ongoing China-Cornell Research Project focusing on the relationship between nutrition and disease, Portman initiated animal studies in which ciwujia was compared with other herbs purported to increase endurance.

When the herb effectively, and safely, outperformed its competition, human trials were started at the Academy of Preventive Medicine in Beijing, as well as at the physiology department at the University of North Texas Health Science Center in Fort Worth.

The Supporting Research

Scientists knew that ciwujia helped ultrafit mountain climbers to reach their physical peaks. Now the researchers wanted to find out how the more typical exerciser, at sea level, could benefit from the herb. After testing ten men on stationary bicycles to measure their muscle power and heart rate, and the levels of lactic acid they produced during a one-hour workout, the subjects were each given 800 mg of ciwujia for the following ten days. Then they were retested.

Dr. Robert Kaman, the director of the exercise physiology lab who conducted the study, observed that:

• There was a significant decrease in the men's average heart rate (147 beats per minute in test number 1, 137 beats per minute in test number 2). This proved that the men had an improved second session that required much less effort than the first one.

• There was a marked decline in the respiratory quotient (RQ), indicating that relatively less energy was produced by carbohydrate metabolism, while there was a considerable, 30 percent, increase in fat metabolism during the cycling hour.

While the specific way in which ciwujia is able to activate fat breakdown and use it as an energy source is not yet understood, it is obvious that its impact on endurance is amazing. Using this ancient herb with modern training techniques can trigger weight loss and boost stamina.

My recommendation for both men and women is to take two 400 mg capsules of Endurox with water twice a day. For best results, it should be taken one to two hours before a training session. If you have a consistent endurance training schedule you should take the capsules daily even on your "rest" days.

Here are the most often questions asked about ciwujia, or Endurox.

1. How does Endurox work?

Endurox alters the way your body fuels your endurance training by shifting the energy source from carbohydrates to fat. This unique carbohydrate-sparing action increases fat metabolism and slows lactic acid buildup, which in turn causes extreme muscle soreness and fatigue. In 1996, a U.S. patent was approved for the use of Endurox to improve exercise performance, raise the metabolism of fat, and delay the accumulation of lactic acid during a workout.

2. How effective is Endurox in metabolizing fat during training?

Studies conducted in the United States and China have shown that Endurox boosts fat metabolism up to 43 percent. Using it can help you reduce body fat while expanding endurance.

3. How useful is Endurox in improving endurance?

The endurance-enhancing properties of Endurox have been studied both in the medical and exercise physiology laboratories. Tests with exercisers have shown that Endurox reduces lactic acid levels up to 33 percent. Additionally, Endurox raises the anaerobic threshold—the ability to exercise maximally up to 12.4 percent—which betters overall workout performance.

4. How useful is Endurox in speeding recovery following a training workout?

Trials conducted in the exercise physiology laboratory revealed that subjects taking Endurox experienced a more rapid decrease in heart rate after working out. Fifteen minutes after training, the heart rate in the Endurox group was 113 percent of the pre-exercise number, versus 135 percent in the control group.

5. Who should not use it?

Endurox can be used safely by all adults.

6. Is Endurox a stimulant or an anabolic steroid?

It is neither one, nor does it prompt side effects associated with either stimulants or anabolic steroids. Endurox, which does not contain caffeine, is marketed in this country by PacificHealth Laboratories.

7. How soon will I feel the benefits of Endurox?

Within three days you should begin to feel a difference. Less soreness following training, as well as an all-around improved workout, are the hallmarks of Endurox use.

8. Where can I purchase Endurox?

Endurox is sold at leading health food stores nationwide.

Endurance Supplement Strategy

Each of the four ergogenics—HMB, creatine, BCAAs, and ciwujia—has been proven to have beneficial and powerful effects on increasing endurance and delaying fatigue. While HMB, creatine, and BCAAs can be used interchangeably, I don't favor one product over another. The decision to use a particular ergogenic is often based on convenience and availability, but the decision to keep using it is based on the results that the ergogenic produces in an individual. All of these products are readily available in leading health food stores and pharmacies nationwide.

To begin, I recommend that you discuss these products with your physician, and then use one product for a minimum of two months. Note the benefits you achieve; if you're satisfied with the gains, you may continue to use it selectively. However, if you want to see if you can achieve similar—or even greater—gains with another product, then

SUMMARY OF THE ERGOGENIC ENHANCERS

Ergogenic Enhancer	What It Does	Daily Recommendation
HMB	Minimizes muscle tissue breakdown; delays onset of fatigue; helps increase muscle size when combined with strength training	3 g: 1 g taken with breakfast, lunch, and dinner.
Creatine	Fuels muscles for short duration, peak performance activities; delays lactic acid production; promotes overall strength gains.	3 g taken with fruit juice at breakfast time or right after training
Branched-chain amino acids (BCAAs)	Synthesizes protein; promotes overal strength gains; helps build muscle; prevents post-workout muscle soreness; delays onset of fatigue.	15 to 20 g in two equal doses. Take one 45–60 minutes prior to exercise the second within 30 minutes of finishing a workout.
Ciwujia (Endurox)	Shifts energy source from carbohydrates to fats during training; slows lactic acid buildup; helps reduce body fat.	Two 400 mg capsules with water one to two hours before training. Take on "rest" days as well.

stop what you are currently taking and begin using another ergogenic for a minimum two-month trial period.

Ciwujia is in a category by itself. It may be taken in combination with any of the other three ergogenics.

When Fatigue Doesn't Go Away

Sometimes, fatigue has causes that go unrecognized. While keeping a killer pace is bound to sap anyone's strength at some point, there are times when debilitating fatigue won't be helped by endurance training or the added push of ergogenic enhancers. In order for you to benefit fully from the Vitality Medicine program, you need to determine whether your fatigue has a medical basis.

Extreme tiredness is not uncommon. At least a quarter of American adults suffer from fatigue that endures for more than two weeks; some feel washed out and run down for six months at a time, or even longer. When a very fatigued patient complains of this particular ailment, there are guidelines I use to determine what might be the underlying cause. I ask:

- when the fatigue occurs, and whether it worsens as the day progresses
- if it disappears after a weekend or vacation, only to return when work begins again
- if the fatigue appeared after the death of a loved one, or another traumatic event
- if the complaint is actually one of physical weakness

In these instances, fatigue is a symptom of a health problem—not overwork, too many personal demands, or any other of a number of external reasons. It is a red flag, and attention must be paid to it. In my experience, prolonged fatigue can be often linked to six major ailments. They are:

- depression
- diabetes

- hepatitis
- iron-deficiency anemia
- sleep deprivation
- thyroid disease

Once diagnosed, there are medical solutions for each condition. But unless they are addressed they can worsen and, in some instances, even become life-threatening. Of course, independent of these six ailments there are other fatigue-causing conditions. Some are linked to rheumatological disorders or to a chronic viral syndrome that triggers fatigue in the muscles, tendons, and ligaments. However, for the most part the six conditions listed above are the most common vitality-sappers that all too often go undiagnosed.

Depression

When Howard, a forty-four-year-old accountant, came to see me, he was engulfed by fatigue.

"The last six months I've been sapped of any energy. I'm so tired all the time that I don't really care about anything— or anybody. I've drifted away from my wife because I feel I have nothing to give her anymore. And I'm too worn out to do anything to help myself."

Struck by the fact that Howard's extreme lethargy was colored by hopelessness, as well as noting other relevant symptoms, I diagnosed his condition as depression. While he had never thought about taking antidepressant drugs, he knew he desperately needed something to help lift him out of his melancholy, and he agreed to take medication.

Three weeks after he started taking his pills, his fatigue started to fade, his spirits began to rise, and he got some of his old energy back. "The terrible truth," he confessed, "was that, before I started taking my medicine, I even contemplated ending my life."

Many of my patients who describe themselves as being chronically fatigued are actually clinically depressed. They are not alone. Major depression may occur in 10 percent of the population, while milder forms can affect as many as 25 percent. Their problem is not imaginary, and telling them, with the best intentions, to get more sleep, pull themselves together, or cheer up is not going to help at all. In fact, it very likely will make them feel worse.

Unfortunately, most depression sufferers receive the wrong treatment or none at all. Often their feelings of self-loathing inhibit them from asking for help. This is a shame, because most of the time their condition has to do with brain chemistry. They either have too much or too little of the brain chemical messengers known as neurotransmitters. Nonchemical causes of depression can include the death of a loved one, marital problems, financial setbacks, or a host of other problems.

Diagnosing depression is not an exact science. However, a major symptom is a change in the way you function. Not being able to take care of "business as usual," being overwhelmed by fatigue and exhaustion, not being interested in sex but feeling hyperemotional, listless in the morning upon awakening, and being tortured by feelings of unworthiness are all characteristics of depression.

Having all of these symptoms for more than two weeks is a sure signal of depression. The good news is that help is readily available. Pharmacological intervention with antidepressant drugs has become the mainstay in treating many cases of acute depression. The newer selective serotonin reuptake inhibitor (SSRI) medications are very effective at decreasing depressive symptoms. They reduce the risk of recurrence and improve a person's overall emotional health. Though family- and work-related problems might require more specialized psychotherapy in addition to the medicine, many people do so well with medications alone that additional help is not required.

Diabetes

At fifty-one, Timothy, a busy airline executive, knew that something was wrong.

"Suddenly I began to feel tired and washed out," he told me. "I haven't been able to shake it for nearly six months and my sex life has all but disappeared. Not only that: I'm urinating much more than usual, and I'm thirsty all the time. And if all this weren't enough, now my vision has suddenly started to change. I can't make out the hands of the kitchen wall clock anymore."

Detecting what I expected Timothy's problem to be—diabetes—was relatively easy. The disclosure about his diminished sex drive, unquenchable thirst, and excess urination were giveaways. The vision problem was another major indicator: It was due to the changes of fluid in his eye lenses, which are classic manifestations of diabetes.

I also asked Timothy to pinch the skin around his navel between his thumb and forefinger. It measured nearly two inches. Men have an increased risk of diabetes if their skinfold thickness is at least one and a quarter inches.

The most definitive answer came from a simple blood sugar exam taken in my office. Normal blood sugar levels are between 70 and 120 mg of glucose per 100 ml of blood. Levels between 140 and 180 put you at a mild risk of complications, and over 200 signifies a moderate risk. Readings over 300 indicate extreme risk. Timothy was lucky: His glucose level was 190.

Just like half of the fourteen million Americans who have Type II diabetes, Timothy wasn't even aware that he had it. Obesity plays a major role in Type II diabetes and, unfortunately, Timothy's weight fit the profile. He carried almost 230 pounds on his five-foot eleven-inch frame, and I informed him immediately that he had to lose thirty-five of them. Cutting back on high-fat foods, and losing weight and maintaining that loss, combined with regular exercise, are the most important components of Type II diabetes therapy. They can bring glucose levels back down to normal. For some people, a half hour of aerobic exercise daily is often enough to clear all the symptoms. However, if diet and exercise are not enough to control glucose levels, then medication is indicated.

To help Timothy lose weight I started him on Redux, chemically known as dexfenfluramine, a powerful appetite-suppressant medication. The drug increases brain levels of the neurotransmitter serotonin, which causes a person to feel full after eating just a few bites of food. An interesting effect of the medication is that it also helps to lower blood glucose levels.

Redux, combined with his daily walking and the 7/20 strength-training program (see page 219), helped pare off Timothy's excess poundage in under three months. With this weight loss came a dramatic drop in his glucose levels as well. Since he now keeps his weight down, avoids fatty foods, and exercises regularly, Timothy has not had any more problems with fatigue—and has kept his diabetes in check.

Hepatitis

Monica came for a checkup after her most recent trip to India. Once a month, the forty-six-year-old textile designer flew out of the country to visit the various mills that printed her fabric. But upon her return she felt so washed out that she couldn't bear the thought of going anywhere, except home to bed.

"International travel has never been a problem for me," she explained. "But since I've come back from this last trip I haven't bounced back from the jet lag the way I usually do. In fact, I've begun to sleep more than ever and, oddly, I'm not hungry. I have to drag myself to work, I'm continually achy, and plowing through the day is really hard. Maybe I picked up some odd strain of flu."

I told Monica that I suspected what she picked up was infectious hepatitis. Many people first mistake hepatitis for the flu, and with good reason. Common symptoms include fatigue, loss of appetite, aching muscles and joints, and fever. While the other symptoms soon disappear, the fatigue can last for months.

Acute viral hepatitis is an inflammation of the liver than can be caused by one of several different viruses. The liver is the body's largest internal organ, and it can be affected by viruses labeled A, B, and C (HCV). Hepatitis D and E are less common in this country. Some forms are benign while others may lead to a chronic infection that can last a lifetime.

Monica had hepatitis A, most likely acquired in a restaurant abroad. This A strain, which can come from poor sanitation and inadequate sewage disposal or contaminated food, water, or utensils, is the most common form of the virus. It is also the most typical kind of hepatitis that Americans contract. Most adults pick it up as Monica did, traveling. Luckily, the virus is relatively harmless and has no lasting effects.

Hepatitis B is usually contracted through sexual contact, contaminated needles, and blood transfusions. About 300,000 new cases are diagnosed each year, with at least eight thousand people dying from related complications, including severe cirrhosis and liver cancer.

Hepatitis C, which is generally transmitted through blood transfusions, is now turning out to be a major health problem. Many times there are no symptoms whatsoever or, if there are, they seem to be flu-like and then disappear quickly. If undetected, the virus often leads to a lifelong infection that can cause cirrhosis of the liver or liver cancer. There is a blood marker for hepatitis C. A liver biopsy may be needed to confirm the extent of the disease.

Laboratory blood tests will identify most hepatitis infections. To date, a high-tech antiviral medication called interferon alpha-2b (Intron) is being used to treat chronic hepatitis B and C.

If you are in a high-risk group (work in the medical field, are a male homosexual, a heterosexual with several partners, or an international traveler to areas where infection rates are high), prevention is the key for reducing your susceptibility. A vaccine is now available for Type A and Type B hepatitis, and you should receive immunization. Three injections are needed for Type B, two for Type A, but both impart long-term immunity. Currently, vaccines are under development for the other forms of the disease.

I gave Monica a series of immunizing vaccinations to protect her from contracting Type B hepatitis again. Her fatigue, though, lasted months before finally dissipating.

Iron-Deficiency Anemia

When Jill came to see me she, like Monica, had also attributed her relentless fatigue to a nasty bout of flu. But months had passed, and the thirty-seven-year-old real estate agent was still exhausted.

"I hate to keep saying it, but I'm so tired all the time. I know I'm working hard, but I always have and I've never felt like this before. I'm so pale—even in the summer. The really scary thing is that I'm breathless and weak. And it's probably silly to mention this at all—but lately I have an insatiable craving to chew on ice cubes. I don't mean the way that most of us do, when we get to the bottom of the iced tea glass and pop a cube to suck on. I mean I keep a glass of ice cubes on my desk and I chew them constantly."

A single parent with two sons in high school, Jill had every excuse to be tired at the end of her day. But she was right: The kind of neverending lassitude that was dragging her down wasn't natural. Her work was suffering, and her relationship with her children was becoming more strained every day.

The ice chewing was an important clue to Jill's condition. So was her pallor, which was a defining sign of iron-deficiency anemia. After confirming that she was not bleeding from any site, I performed a simple blood test to check her ferritin levels. The results confirmed my suspicion that she was, indeed, anemic. The amount of iron in her blood was much lower than it should have been, which was causing her troubling symptoms.

In cases like these the solution is simple: Add iron-rich foods to your diet along with daily iron supplements. The best sources of dietary heme iron—the type most readily absorbed by the body—include meat, poultry, and fish. Iron-enriched breads and cereals will help as well, especially if they are eaten along with sources of vitamin C. Iron absorption is greatly increased in the presence of this vitamin. Remember: Supplementation is necessary to heal iron-deficiency anemia; food alone will not have the desired effect.

Much relieved, Jill followed my recommendations for an iron-rich diet and took her supplements. Three weeks later another blood test was done to check her iron levels. At that point the dosage of her supplements was adjusted; the rate of iron absorption decreases as levels rise. The supplements were continued for an additional two months after her blood tests returned to normal—as did her life.

Note: Women must be especially vigilant about their iron intake, especially women of child-bearing age. Menstrual bleeding is a major cause of iron deficiency and can quickly lead to anemia. This means that your blood doesn't have enough hemoglobin, which carries oxygen to your cells. Iron-deficiency anemia is a very common problem for women in their premenopausal period: It affects at least 20 percent of forty-five-year-old women. If the woman is an active exerciser or vegetarian, the percentage is even higher. Iron deficiency in men is less common and is typically caused by blood loss from internal hemorrhoids or a more serious bleeding malignancy in the colon.

Sleep Deprivation

Charles arrived at my office with one thing on his mind: He was tired and lacking energy. The cause was easy to trace: the hours of his new job.

"I just switched jobs on Wall Street," he told me. "One of my new responsibilities includes tracking Asian stocks and business transactions as well as handling the stock-related business coming from Japan. Every night I go to bed at 10:00 P.M. or so and have to wake up at 3:00 A.M. so that I can go to my den, check my computer, and start calling Tokyo. Then I leave for the downtown office at 5:30 A.M. I guess the days of eight-hours-a-night sleep are gone forever. I've been doing this for only a month—and I feel like my whole life is unraveling."

It wasn't surprising he was so tired. Charles was suffering from sleep deprivation. Our bodies crave sleep, and don't allow for much tampering with it. Try to deprive yourself of it—or if you suffer from insomnia—and you're going to pay with poor job performance, a suppressed immune system, and the potential for a serious accident because you can't be as sharp-minded and alert as you need to be.

Working at cross-purposes to his circadian rhythms proved to be more difficult than Charles knew. After one week on the job, he had accumulated a "sleep debt" of ten hours. He felt out of sorts, his muscles were rubbery, and he ached in places that had never before bothered him. He caught a cold. But most disturbing was his absentmindedness, which caused him great embarrassment at work.

His home life wasn't much better. Irritable and argumentative, he routinely started to fall asleep before dinner. He tried to get more sleep on the weekends, but even after an extra ten hours of sleep he still felt groggy and out of sorts.

Since Charles had no physical problems, I recommended some major changes that would help to erase his daytime drowsiness and restore his sleep/wake cycle. I told him he had to get at least seven hours of sleep a night, which meant getting to bed no later than 8:00 P.M., and distractions like the phone had to be eliminated from his bedroom. I recommended that he install dark window shades in the bedroom to screen out streetlights and other intrusions, and more powerful lighting in the home office. When he went to his den to work, snapping on the bright lights would halt the production of melatonin, sending a signal to the brain that the sleep cycle is over and that it's definitely time to wake up.

Charles called me the next day to say that he had followed my directions and had slept very well the night before. Two weeks later he reported that he was wide awake every day at work, and his sleep was back to normal.

Sleep rests and restores your body. During this cycle, growth hormone is released which helps renew body tissues and form new red blood cells. Researchers have also found that deep sleep helps the body mobilize its defenses against illness.

While each of us has a unique sleep pattern, our individual minimum requirement is unyielding. Whether it is four or ten hours a night—most adults need anywhere from seven to nine—we need sleep to rejuvenate ourselves mentally. The bottom line on how much sleep you need is marked by knowing how many hours you need to feel alert and rested the next day. When you sleep well, you're more creative, productive, and sociable.

Thyroid Disease

Justine was the typical on-the-go sort of person. If she wasn't doing more than two things at once she felt that she was slacking off. But when the office manager reached the age of forty-seven, she began to notice some gradual changes that brought her to my office.

"My muscles hurt, I'm tired, and for the first time my periods are lasting a longer time, and the flow is much heavier. I'm also gaining weight. I know I'm perimenopausal so I can rationalize these changes. But what is really troubling me is that I'm having trouble climbing two flights of stairs to my office. Frankly, I'm getting scared," she said.

I suggested a simple, reliable blood test that measures TSH (thyroid-stimulating hormone). It pinpoints the thyroid trouble at once—even if a person doesn't have any symptoms. I perform it regularly on my patients who are over forty. It revealed that Justine's TSH levels were high; she had an underactive thyroid, or hypothyroidism. I started her on hormone-replacement therapy with a synthetic form of thyroxine, the thyroid hormone that her body was no longer producing naturally. Within a week she felt better and after a few months all of her symptoms were gone.

The thyroid gland produces the hormones that regulate your metabolic system and muscle strength. Small, with the appearance of a bow tie, the thyroid wraps around the windpipe just below the Adam's apple. It extracts iodine from the blood and produces thyroxine and triiodothyronine, two hormones that orchestrate the body's metabolic functioning.

Thyroid disease develops when your thyroid gland begins to malfunction, changing its normal output of hormone. Too little, and you have hypothyroidism. Too much, and you have hyperthyroidism. Hypothyroidism is twice as prevalent as hyperthyroidism. Both ailments can cause extreme fatigue.

An underactive thyroid affects upward of 11 million Americans; half don't even know they have it. Women are four times as prone as men to have this problem—females over the age of forty are most likely to be affected. The condition is most probably attributable to an immune system malfunction in which the thyroid gland is attacked by the body's own antibodies. Vague symptoms of fatigue and forgetfulness, mood swings, as well as unexpected weight gain, are common symptoms. Chalked up to overwork and stress, these markers are often ignored by people who have them. Consequently, they don't do anything about them and, unfortunately, the symptoms persist and get worse.

Harold, a fifty-three-year-old television producer, was diagnosed with the other type of thyroid malfunction: hyperthyroidism, or Graves' disease, which is marked by low TSH levels. Though he was uncommonly agitated, he nevertheless found himself counting the hours at work before he could get home to bed. This was due to the extra-large doses of hormone his thyroid produced that were toxic to muscles and triggered great fatigue. I prescribed a medication to slow down his hormone production. (The ailment can also be treated with radioactive iodine followed by thyroid hormones.) In a few weeks, he was feeling fine again.

In both Justine's and Harold's cases, annual TSH tests are performed to make sure that dosages are at their proper levels.

How Healthy Are You?

Vitality Medicine starts with a good physical exam. The initial oral history your doctor takes is a critical component in assessing your overall health. I start my exams with a detailed question-and-answer investigation that covers personal background, employment, daily nutrition, and exercise habits, as well as past medical history. I start with a review of systems in which I ask about the functioning of body parts and organ systems. These include eyes, ears, throat, heart, bowels, reflexes, skin, muscles, joints, and bones. I inquire about the person's emotional health, marital or relationship life, and sexual health. Of course I measure height and weight, too. Then I review the family medical tree.

Even if you feel perfectly fine, a comprehensive physical

exam can detect unsuspected conditions. High blood pressure and diabetes, both of which can be controlled with medication, as well as curable cancers of the breast, cervix, colon, and prostate, can be detected before symptoms arise and complications develop.

Acute illness may only give a brief warning before it strikes with full force. Unfortunately, most often we don't have any advance warning before a serious illness manifests itself. Any foreknowledge of a potentially health-threatening condition is a critical ally of Vitality Medicine.

The physical exam that I give my patients screens for all signs of disease. More specifically, however, it gives me an accurate assessment of their current health status. Typically, I recommend the physical to establish a primary baseline, as well as a starting point for my overall vitality program. A periodic reevaluation at least once a year is necessary.

Once the traditional history, review of systems, physical exam, and laboratory tests have been completed and reviewed, I then initiate the Vitality Medicine component of my program, with specific emphasis on memory, sexuality, appearance, antioxidant status, cardio-protection, and endurance.

The Vitality Medicine Goal

Becoming the best you can be—mentally, physically, and emotionally—is what I consider to be our life's best work. To fully maximize these potentials, I feel that we are meant to be "works in progress." Building on our strengths and enhancing our skills are the hallmarks of people living their lives fully. Endurance is the key that opens the doors to unlimited possibilities.

Afterword

Vitality Medicine offers you the keys to adding years of peak performance to your life. We now have the means to remain vital longer than any other generation in history. The choice is truly yours. All you need is the motivation and a physician who will work with you—a doctor willing to help you kick away all the conventional notions of aging and the stereotypes of middle age, a partner and "coach" in helping you gain access to every means available to you to redesign, reinvent, and rejuvenate yourself in order to be **YOUNGER AT LAST.**

Be well, my friends.

Bibliography

The following references represent the significant technical and scientific books and articles that have been used as source material. They are grouped according to topic.

Memory

Acetylcholine:
Dunant, Y., and M. Israel. "The Release of Acetylcholine." *Scientific American* 252 (4): 58–67 (1985).

Caffeine:
Loke, W. "Effects of Caffeine on Mood and Memory." *Physiology and Behavior* (44): 367–72 (1988).

Deprenyl:
Arnsten, A., J. Cai, B. Murphy, *et al.* "Dopamine D1 Receptor Mechanisms in the Cognitive Performance of Young Adults and Aged Monkeys." *Psychopharmacology* (116): 143–51 (1994).

Knoll, J. "Deprenyl medication: A Strategy to Modulate the Age-Related Decline of the Striatal Dopaminergic System." *Journal of the American Geriatric Society* 40(8): 839–47 (August 1992).

———. "The Pharmacology of Selegiline." *Acta Neurologica Scandinavica* (126): 83–91 (1989).

———. "The Possible Mechanism of Action of Deprenyl

Bibliography

in Parkinson's Disease." *Journal of Neural Transmission* (43): 239–44 (1978).

————. "Extension of Life Span of Rats by Long-term Deprenyl Treatment." *Mount Sinai Journal of Medicine* (55): 67–74 (1988).

Exercise:

"Exercise Can Go to Your Head: Working Out May Make You Happier, Smarter, and More Creative." *Consumer Reports on Health* (vol. 7, no. 9): 104 (Sept. 1995).

Food:

Algeri, S. "Potential Strategies Against Age-Related Brain Deterioration: Dietary and Pharmacological Approaches." *Annals of New York Academy of Science* (663): 376–83 (1992).

Benton, D., and G. Roberts. "Effect of Vitamin and Mineral Supplementation on Intelligence of a Sample of Schoolchildren." *The Lancet* 140–43 (Jan. 23, 1988).

Greenwood, C. "The Role of Diet in Modulating Brain Metabolism and Behavior." *Contemporary Nutrition* 14, no. 7 (1989).

Ginkgo biloba:

Allain, H. "Effect of Two Doses of *Ginkgo biloba* Extract on the Dual-Coding Test in Elderly Subjects." *Clinical Therapeutics* (3): 549–58 (May–June 1993).

Kleijen, J., and P. Knipschild. "*Ginkgo biloba* for Cerebral Insufficiency." *British Journal of Clinical Pharmacology* (34): 352–58 (1992).

Hydergine:

Exton-Smith, A., *et al.* "Clinical Experience with Ergot Alkaloids." *Aging* 23 (1983).

Emmenegger, H., and W. Meier-Ruge. "The Actions of Hydergine on the Brain." *Pharmacology* (1): 65–78 (1968).

Hughes, J., *et al.* "An Ergot Alkaloid Preparation (Hydergine) in the Treatment of Dementia: A Critical Review of the Clinical Literature." *Journal of the American Geriatrics Society* (24) 490–97 (1976).

Spiegel, R., *et al.* "A Controlled Long-term Study with Ergoloid Mesylates (Hydergine) in Healthy, Elderly Volunteers: Results After Three Years." *Journal of the Geriatrics Society* (vol. 31, no. 9): 549–55 (1983).

Weil, C., ed. "Pharmacology and Clinical Pharmacology of Hydergine." *Handbook of Experimental Pharmacology.* New York: Springer-Verlag, 1978.

Nicotine:

Krebs, S. "Effects of Smoking on Memory for Prose Passages." *Physiological Behavior* (Suppl. 4): 723–27 (Oct. 1994).

Van Duijin, C., and A. Hofman. "Relation Between Nicotine Intake and Alzheimer's Disease." *British Medical Journal* (vol. 302, no. 6791): 1491–94 (June 22, 1991).

Phosphatidylserine:

Amaducci, L., T. Crook, *et al.* "Use of Phosphatidylserine in Alzheimer's Disease." *Annals of New York Academy of Science* (640): 245–49 (1991).

Crook, T. "Effects of Phosphatidylserine in Age-Associated Memory Impairment." *Neurology* (vol. 41, no. 5): 644–49 (May 1991).

Crook, T., and W. Petrie. "Effects of Phosphatidylserine in Alzheimer's Disease." *Psychopharmacology Bulletin* (28): 61–66 (1992).

Klinkhammer, P., and B. Szelies. "Effect of Phosphatidylserine on Cerebral Glucose Metabolism in Alzheimer's Disease." *Dementia* (1): 197–201 (1990).

Monteleone, P., L. Beinat, *et al.* "Effects of Phosphatidylserine on the Neuroendocrine Response to Physical Stress in Humans." *Neuroendocrinology* (52): 243–48 (1990).

Vitamin supplementation:

Benton, D., *et al.* "The Impact of Long-term Vitamin Supplementation on Cognitive Functioning." *Psychopharmacology* (117): 298–305 (1995).

Guilarte, T. "Vitamin B_6 and Cognitive Development: Recent Research Findings from Human and Animal Studies." *Nutrition Review* (51): 193–98 (1993).

Bibliography

Sexual Performance

Abel, E. *Psychoactive Drugs and Sex.* New York: Plenum Press, 1985.

Anand, M., *The Art of Sexual Ecstasy.* Los Angeles: Jeremy P. Tarcher, 1989.

Bansal, S. "Sexual Dysfunction in Hypertensive Men: A Critical Review of the Literature." *Hypertension* (12): 1–10 (1988).

Buffum, J. "Pharmacosexology: The Effects of Drugs on Sexual Function." *Journal of Psychoactive Drugs* (14): 5–44 (1982).

Crawford, D. "Organic Causes of Male Sexual Dysfunction: The Evaluation and Treatment of Impotence." *Modern Medicine* (Sept. 1991).

Crowe, L., and W. George. "Alcohol and Human Sexuality: Review and Integration." *Psychology Bulletin* (105): 374–86 (1989).

Gessa, G. "Role of Serotonin and Dopamine in Male Sexual Behavior." In *Sexual Behavior: Pharmacology and Biochemistry.* New York: Raven Press, 1975.

Herman, J., A. Brotman, *et al.* "Fluoxetine-Induced Sexual Dysfunction." *Journal of Clinical Psychiatry* (51): 25–27 (1990).

Rosen, R., and A. Ashton. "Prosexual Drugs: Empirical Status of the 'New Aphrodisiacs.'" *Archives of Sexual Behavior* 22 (6): 521–43 (1993).

Stevenson, R., and L. Solyom. "The Aphrodisiac Effect of Fenfluramine: Two Case Reports of a Possible Side Effect to the Use." *Journal of Clinical Psychiatry* (10): 69–71 (1990).

Yager, J. "Bethanechol Chloride Can Reverse Erectile and Ejaculatory Dysfunction Induced by Tricyclic Antidepressants and Mazindol: Case Report." *Journal of Clinical Psychiatry* (47): 210–11 (1986).

Deprenyl:

Dallo, J., and J. Knoll. "The Aphrodisiac Effect of Deprenyl in Male Rats." *Acta Physiologica Hungarica,* 75 Suppl. (1990).

Knoll, L. "The Pharmacology of Selegiline (-) Deprenyl:

New Aspects." *Acta Neurologica Scandinavica* (126): 83–91 (1989).

Nitric oxide:
Snyder, S., and D. Bredt. "Biological Roles of Nitric Oxide." *Scientific American* (May 1992).

Trazodone:
Gartrell, N. "Increased Libido in Women Receiving Trazodone." *American Journal of Psychiatry* (143): 781–82 (1986).
Lal, S., O. Rios, *et al.* "Treatment of Impotence with Trazodone: A Case Report." *Journal of Urology* (143): 819–20 (1990).

Wellbutrin:
Feighner, J., *et al.* "Double-Blind Comparison of Bupropion and Fluoxetine in Depressed Outpatients." *Journal of Clinical Psychiatry* (52): 329–35 (1991).

Yohimbe:
Clark, J., E. Smith, *et al.* "Enhancement of Sexual Motivation in Male Rats by Yohimbine." *Science* (225): 847–49 (1984).
Thiebolt, L., and J. Berthelay. "Preventive and Curative Action of a Bark Extract from an African Plant, Pygeym Africanum, on Experimental Prostatic Adenoma." *Therapie* (26): 575–80 (1971).

Image

Darr, D., S. Combs, S. Dunston, *et al.* "Topical Vitamin C Protects Porcine Skin from Ultraviolet Radiation-Induced Damage." *British Journal of Dermatology* (127): 247–53 (1992).
Gershoff, S. "Vitamin C (Ascorbic Acid): New Roles, New Requirements?" *Nutrition Review* (51): 313–26 (1993).

Pycnogenol

Angier, N. "Free Radicals: The Price We Pay for Breathing." *New York Times Magazine,* Apr. 25, 1993, 62 ff.

Bibliography

Fuhrman, B., A. Levy, *et al.* "Consumption of Red Wine with Meals Reduces the Susceptibility of Human Plasm and Low-Density Lipoprotein to Lipid Peroxidation." *American Journal of Clinical Nutrition* (61): 549–54 (1995).

Gaziano, J., J. Burning, *et al.* "Dietary Antioxidants and Cardiovascular Disease." *Annals of the New York Academy of Science* (669): 249–59 (1992).

Harman, D. "Free Radical Theory of Aging: Nutritional Implications." *Age* (1): 143–50 (1978).

Hertog, M. "Dietary Antioxidant Flavonoids and the Risk of Coronary Heart Disease: The Zutphen Elderly Study." *The Lancet* (342): 1007–11 (1993).

Masquelier, J., J. Michaud, *et al.* "Flavanoids and Pycnogenols." *International Journal for Vitamin and Nutrition Research* 49 (3): 307–11 (1979).

Tixier, J., G. Godeau, *et al.* "Evidence in Vivo and In Vitro Studies That Binding of Pycnogenols to Elastin Affects Its Rate of Degradation by Elastases." *Biochemical Pharmacology* (vol. 33, no. 24): 3933–39 (1984).

Yongqi, R., L. Lin, *et al.* "Pycnogenol Protects Vascular Endothelial Cells from T-Butyl Hydroperoxide-Induced Oxidant Injury." *Biotechnology Therapeutics* 5 (3 & 4): 117–26 (1994–95).

Heart Protection

CoQ10:

Baggio, E. "Italian Multicenter Study on the Safety and Efficacy of Coenzyme Q10 as Adjunctive Therapy in Heart Failure." *Clinical Investigator* (71): S145–49 (1993).

Bliznakov, E. *The Miracle Nutrient Coenzyme Q10.* New York: Bantam Books, 1986.

Folkers, K. "Heart Failure Is a Dominant Deficiency of Coenzyme A10 and Challenges for Future Clinical Research on CoQ10." *Clinical Investigator* (71 8 Suppl.): S51–54 (1993).

————. "Therapy with Coenzyme Q10 of Patients in Heart Failure Who Are Eligible or Ineligible for Transplant." *Biochemical and Biophysical Research Communications* (182, 1): 247–53 (January 15, 1992).

Bibliography

Greenberg, S. "Co-enzyme Q10: A New Drug for Cardiovascular Disease." *Journal of Clinical Pharmacology* (30, 7): 596–608 (1990).

Lansjoen, P. "Isolated Diastolic Dysfunction of the Myocardium and Its Response to CoQ-10 Treatment." *Clinical Investigator* (71, 8 Suppl.): S140–42 (1993).

Menopause:

Bachman, G. "The Changes Before 'the Change': Strategies for the Transition to the Menopause." *Postgraduate Medicine* 95 (4): 113–15 (Mar. 1994).

Belchetz, P. "Hormonal Treatment of Postmenopausal Women." *New England Journal of Medicine* 330 (15): 1062–71 (Apr. 14, 1994).

Gambrell, R. D., Jr. "Update on Hormone Replacement Therapy." *American Family Physician* 46 (5 Suppl.): 87S–96S (Nov. 1992).

Griffing, G., and S. H. Allen. "Estrogen Replacement Therapy at Menopause: How Benefits Outweigh Risks." *Postgraduate Medicine* 96 (5): 131–40 (Oct. 1994).

Osteoporosis:

Allen, S. H., "Primary Osteoporosis: Methods to Combat Bone Loss That Accompanies Aging." *Postgraduate Medicine* 93 (8): 43–46, 49–50, 53–55 (June 1993).

Dawson–Hughes, B., P. F. Jacques, and C. N. Shnipp. "Dietary Calcium Intake and Bone Loss from the Spine in Healthy Postmenopausal Women." *American Journal of Clinical Nutrition* 46 (1987), 68–87.

Isenbarger, D., and B. Chapin. "Osteoporosis: Current Pharmacologic Options for Prevention and Treatment." *Postgraduate Medicine* (101 N. 1): 129–41 (Jan. 1997).

Johnston, C. D., C. W. Slemenda, and J. L. Melton III. "Clinical Use of Bone Densitometry." *New England Journal of Medicine* 374: 1105–9 (1991).

Lieberman, U., and S. Weiss. "Effect of Oral Alendronate on Bone Mineral Density and the Incidence of Fractures in Postmenopausal Osteoporosis." *New England Journal of Medicine*, 333 (22): 1437–43 (1995).

"NIH Consensus Development on Optimal Calcium Intake." *Journal of the American Medical Association* (272): 1942–48 (1994).

Riggs, B. L. "Overview of Osteoporosis." *Western Journal of Medicine* 154 (1): 63–77 (Jan. 1991).

Wardlaw, G. M. "Putting Osteoporosis in Perspective." *Journal of the American Dietetic Association* 93 (9): 1000–6 (Sept. 1993).

Statin medication:

Davidson, M., *et al.* "The Efficacy of Six-Week Tolerability of Simvastatin 80 and 160 mg/day." *American Journal of Cardiology* 79 (1): 38–42 (Jan. 1, 1997).

Pitt, R., *et al.* "Provastatin Limitation of Atherosclerosis in the Coronary Arteries (PLAC I): Reduction in Atherosclerosis Progression and Clinical Events." *Journal of the American College of Cardiology* (26): 1133–39 (1995).

Stress:

Tavris, C. *Anger: The Misunderstood Emotion.* Rev. ed. New York: Simon and Schuster, 1989.

Williams, R. *The Trusting Heart: Great News About Type A Behavior.* New York: Times Books/Random House, 1989.

Ultrafast CT:

Budoff, M., *et al.* "Ultrafast Computed Tomography as a Diagnostic Modality in the Detection of Coronary Artery Disease: A Multicenter Study." *Circulation* (93): 898–904 (1996).

Guerci, A., L. Spandaro, J. Popma, *et al.* "Relation of Coronary Calcium Score by Electron Beam Computed Tomography to Arteriographic Findings in Asymptomatic and Symptomatic Adults." *American Journal of Cardiology* 79 (2): 128–33 (Jan. 15, 1997).

Kaufmann, R. B., P. A. Peyser, *et al.* "Quantification of Coronary Artery Calcium by Electron Beam Computed Tomography for Determination of Severity of Angiographic Coronary Artery Disease in Younger Patients." *Journal of the American College of Cardiology* (25): 626–32 (1995).

Bibliography

Rumberger, J., P. A. Sheedy, *et al.* "Coronary Calcium, as Determined by Electron Beam Computed Tomography, and Coronary Artery Disease on Arteriogram: Effect of Patient's Sex on Diagnosis." *Circulation* (91): 1363–67 (1995).

Vitamins:

Abbey, M., and P. Nestel. "Antioxidant Vitamins and Low-Density Lipoprotein Oxidation." *American Journal of Clinical Nutrition* (58): 525–32 (1993).

Carethers, M. "Diagnosing Vitamin B_{12} Deficiency, a Common Geriatric Disorder." *Geriatrics* (43, 3): 89–94, 105–7, 111–12 (1988).

Chasan-Tabar, L., J. Selhub, I. Rosenberg, *et al.* "Prospective Study of Folate and Vitamin B_6 and Risk of Myocardial Infarction." *American Journal of Epidemiology* (138): 603 (1993).

Deijen, J., E. van der Beek, *et al.* "Vitamin B_6 Supplementation in Elderly Men: Effects on Mood, Memory, Performance and Mental Effort." *Psychopharmacology* (109): 489–96 (1992).

Dyckener, T., and P. Wester. "Effects of Magnesium on Blood Pressure." *British Medical Journal* (286): 1847 (1983).

Jialal, I., and S. Grundy. "Effect of Combined Supplementation with Alpha-tocopherol, Ascorbate, and Beta Carotene on Low-Density Lipoprotein Oxidation." *Circulation* (88): 2780–86 (1993).

Kok, F., J. Schrijver, A. Hofman, *et al.* "Low Vitamin B_6 Status in Patients with Acute Myocardial Infarction." *American Journal of Cardiology* (63): 513–16 (1989).

Morgan, K., G. Stampley, *et al.* "Magnesium and Calcium Dietary Intakes of the U.S. Population." *Journal of the American College of Nutrition* (4): 195–206 (1985).

Omaye, S. "An Overview of Vitamin E Deficiency in Humans: Part I." *Nutrition Reports* (11): 17, 24 (1993).

Robinson, K., E. Mayer, and W. Jacobsen. "Homocysteine and Coronary Artery Disease." *Cleveland Clinic Journal of Medicine* (61): 438–50 (1994).

Prasad, K., and J. Kaira. "Oxygen Free Radicals and Hypercholesterolemic Atherosclerosis: Effect of Vitamin E." *American Heart Journal* (125): 958–73 (1991).

Selhub, J. "Vitamin Status and Intake as Primary Determinants of Homocysteinemia in Elderly Population." *Journal of the American Medical Association* (270): 2693–98 (1993).

Stampfer, M., and W. Willett. "Homocysteine and Marginal Vitamin Deficiency." *Journal of the American Medical Association* (270): 2726–27 (1993).

Stampfer, M., and M. Malinow. "Can Lowering Homocysteine Levels Reduce Cardiovascular Risk?" *New England Journal of Medicine* (332, 5): 328 (Feb. 2, 1995).

Women:

Barry, P. "Coronary Artery Disease in Older Women." *Geriatrics* 48 (Suppl. 1): 4–8 (June 1993).

Eaker, E. D., J. Pinsky, and W. P. Castelli. "Myocardial Infarction and Coronary Death Among Women: Psychosocial Predictors from a 20-year Follow-up of Women in the Framingham Study." *American Journal of Epidemiology* 135 (8): 854–64 (Apr. 15, 1992).

Eaker, E. D., J. H. Chesebro, *et al.* "Cardiovascular Disease in Women." *Circulation* 88 (4, pt. 1): 1999–2009 (Oct. 1993).

Kostis, J. B., A. C. Wilson, K. O'Dowd, *et al.* "Sex Differences in the Management and Long-term Outcome of Acute Myocardial Infarction: A Statewide Study" (MIDAS Study Group; Myocardial Infarction Data Acquisition System). *Circulation* 90 (4): 1715–30 (Oct. 1994).

Stampfer, M., G. Colditz, *et al.* "Postmenopausal Estrogen Therapy and Cardiovascular Disease: Ten-year Follow-up from the Nurses' Health Study." *New England Journal of Medicine* (325, 11): 756–62 (1991).

Endurance

BCAAs:

Bloomstrand, E., P. Hassmen, B. Ekblom, *et al.* "Administration of Branched-Chain Amino Acids During Sustained Exercise: Effects on Performance and on Plasma

Concentration of Some Amino Acids." *International Journal of Sports Nutrition* (2): 191–95 (1992).

Blomstrand, E., and E. Newsholme. "Effect of Branched-Chain Amino Acid Supplementation on the Exercise-Induced Change in Aromatic Amino Acid Concentration in Human Muscle." *Acta Physiologica Scandinavica* (146): 293–98 (1992).

Butterfield, G. "Amino Acids and High Protein Diets." In *Perspectives in Exercise Science and Sports Medicine* (vol. 4, Chap. 3), *Ergogenics: Enhancement of Performance in Exercise and Sport,* D. R. Lamb and M. Williams, eds. Dubuque, Iowa: Wm. C. Brown Publishers, 1991. 87–122.

Carli, G. "Changes in the Exercise-Induced Hormone Response to Branched-Chain Amino Acid Administration." *European Journal of Applied Physiology* (64): 272–77 (1992).

Fenstrom, J. "Dietary Amino Acids and Brain Function." *Journal of the American Dietitic Association* (94): 71–77 (1994).

MacLean, D., and T. Graham. "Stimulation of Muscle Ammonia Production During Exercise Following Branched-Chain Amino Acid Supplementation in Humans." *Journal of Physiology* (493, 3): 909–22 (1996).

Creatine:

Earnest, C., and Snell, P. "The Effect of Creatine Monohydrate Ingestion on Anaerobic Power Indices, Muscular Strength and Body Composition." *Acta Physiologica Scandinavica* (1153, 2): 207–9 (Feb. 1995).

Gordon, A., E. Hultman, *et al.* "Creatine Supplementation in Chronic Heart Failure Increases Skeletal Muscle Creatine Phosphate and Muscle Performance." (30, 3): 413–18 (Sept. 30, 1995).

Greenhaff, P. "Creatine and Its Application as an Ergogenic Aid." *International Journal of Sports Nutrition* (5, Suppl.): S100–10 (June 1995).

Maughan, R. "Creatine Supplementation and Exercise Performance." *International Journal of Sports Nutrition* (5, 2): 94–101 (June 1995).

Bibliography

Exercise:

Seals, D., J. M. Hagberb, B. F. Hurley, *et al.* "Endurance Training in Older Men and Women, 1: Cardiovascular Responses to Exercise." *Journal of Applied Physiology* (57): 1024–29 (1984).

Streja, D., and D. Mymin. "Moderate Exercise and High-Density Lipoprotein Cholesterol." *Journal of the American Medical Association* (243): 2190–92 (1979).

Whitehouse, F. "Motivation for Fitness." *Guide to Fitness After 50.* Dr. Raymond Harris and Lawrence J. Frankel, eds. New York: Plenum, 1977. 171–89.

HMB:

Nissen, S., R. Sharp, *et al.* "The Effect of Leucine Metabolite b-Hydroxy-b-Methyl Butyrate on Muscle Metabolism During Resistance-Exercise Training (forthcoming, *American Journal of Applied Physiology*).

Nissen, S., and D. Webb. Analysis of b-Hydroxy-b-Methyl Butyrate in Plasma by Gas Chromatography and Mass Spectrometry." *Annals of Biochemistry* (188): 17–19 (1990).

Nissen, S., R. Wilhelm, and J. C. Fuller. "Effect of b-Hydroxy-b-Methylbutyrate (HMB) Supplementation on Strength and Body Composition of Trained and Untrained Males Undergoing Intense Resistance Training." *Experimental Biology 1996 Conference Presentation Abstract* (1996).

Testosterone:

Bhasin, S., T. Storer, *et al.* "The Effects of Supraphysiologic Doses of Testosterone on Muscle Size and Strength in Normal Men." *New England Journal of Medicine* (335): 1–7 (July 4, 1996).

Acknowledgments

WRITING THIS BOOK brought together many people who supported and helped us along the way. Again, to Nancy and Herb Katz, our literary agents, our deepest gratitude for patiently guiding and encouraging us at each step. Their enthusiasm, motivation, and inspiration are deeply appreciated. We could not have completed this work without their able assistance, for which we are most grateful.

Our deep thanks go to Susan Suffes for her thoughtful attention, insightful comments, and invaluable contributions to the organization, reviewing, and shaping of the manuscript. We could not have done it without her ongoing support.

Special thanks and appreciation to our editor, Fred Hills, for his invaluable suggestions and keen understanding of our purpose; and thanks as well to publisher Carolyn Reidy and associate publisher Michele Martin, who believed in the importance of our message. And to Hilary Black, thanks for all her confidence and helpful editorial suggestions.

Barry Zide, M.D., a friend and colleague, once again offered his time and astute observations in manuscript preparation, as well as other helpful comments and advice. We would also like to thank Charles Anderson, M.D., for his

Acknowledgments

support and expertise in alternative and complementary medicine techniques, and Wojciech Palka, M.D., senior resident at Lenox Hill Hospital, for his enthusiasm and assistance in gathering information on a wide variety of subjects.

Our gratitude is also extended to those colleagues who took time from their busy schedules to offer helpful comments and advice on the complex estrogen pathways and the appropriate use of hormones: Frederick Naftolin, M.D., Ph.D.; Lyla Nachtigall, M.D.; Leon Lewenstein, M.D.; and Mary Wilson, M.D.

Our special thanks are extended to Nathalie Guitay, Thierry Philippe, Michel Van Welden, Kathleen Appell, and Michael Sands of LPG USA for their assistance and support with Endermologie. Thanks, too, to Charles LeRoy, M.D., and his wife Gail, good friends and colleagues who alerted us to this remarkable technique, and Paula Moynahan, M.D., for her support in the Endermologie project. Also, to Carmel Donovan, M.D., for her participation in our cellulite study, and to Robert Ersek, M.D., for his insights on cellulite. Our heartfelt thanks to Jeannette Graf, M.D., for her tremendous vitality and knowledge in the field of cosmeceuticals, and to Simon Erani for his ongoing assistance in this cutting-edge area.

Our warm thanks to Alan Guerci, M.D., for detailing the intricacies of the Ultrafast CT. For their insights into the Cardiophone and the future of telemedicine, our thanks to David Galbut, M.D., Abraham Galbut, Yaniv Dagan, and David Bluth. For their insights into cardiac patient monitoring, our thanks to Alan Spiegel, M.D., and Kenneth Krauss, M.D. And to the late Peter Pasternack, M.D., for his support, vision, and friendship. He is deeply missed.

When it came to our work with ergogenics, particularly branched-chain amino acids, Francesco Dioguardi, M.D., was always there with advice and help.

Thanks, too, to Sam Kirchner, Ph.D., and Scott Wetzler, Ph.D., for their help with stress- and anger-reduction strategies.

We are also grateful to the following for their help with various parts of the book: Robert Portman, Ph.D., Steven Nissen, D.V.M.; Naji Abumrad, M.D.; Ronald Watson,

Acknowledgments

Ph.D.; Rob Rideout and his staff at MicroFit; Lance Goodemann; Wei Jiang, M.D.; Jeffrey Glasser, M.D.; Michael and Denise Margulies of Med Fitness; Michael Buckner, Ph.D.; Roy Geronemus, M.D.; Carl Harris; Mark Sherry; David Bank, M.D.; Timothy McInerney; Richard Wurtman, M.D.; Paul Spiers, Ph.D.; Wayne Meyers, M.D.; Russ Mandor, D.D.S., and his wife, Tanya; Lindsay Rosenwald, M.D.; and Russell Gellis. Thanks, too, to Charles Kaner, D.D.S.; Seema Boesky; Sandy Frucher; Ben Lambert; Ari Genger; John Hunter, M.D.; Louis Marx; Roger Deutsch, M.D.; Bill Beslow; Greg Katz; John Deats, Tony Kovner, David Neiman, and Dr. John Brademas for their good counsel. And of course, to Jack Simpson, for his very discerning and critical eye.

Thanks to our illustrator, Timothy Jeffs, and to Dr. Lamm's entire office staff—Alicia Nation, Grace Grabowska, Deborah Aviles, and Eva Martinez—who helped pitch in and manage patient responsibilities so time could be found during the day to work on the text. And to Charles Maltz, M.D., for all of his kind efforts and assistance.

We would also like to gratefully acknowledge Dr. Lamm's patients, whose experiences in Vitality Medicine are the foundation of this book. Thank you for allowing us to share your stories and spread the exciting news about Vitality Medicine to a national audience.

Index

Index

Index

Index

Index

Index

Index

Index

Index

Index